AF552631

HAIR STORIES

ROHINA HOFFMAN

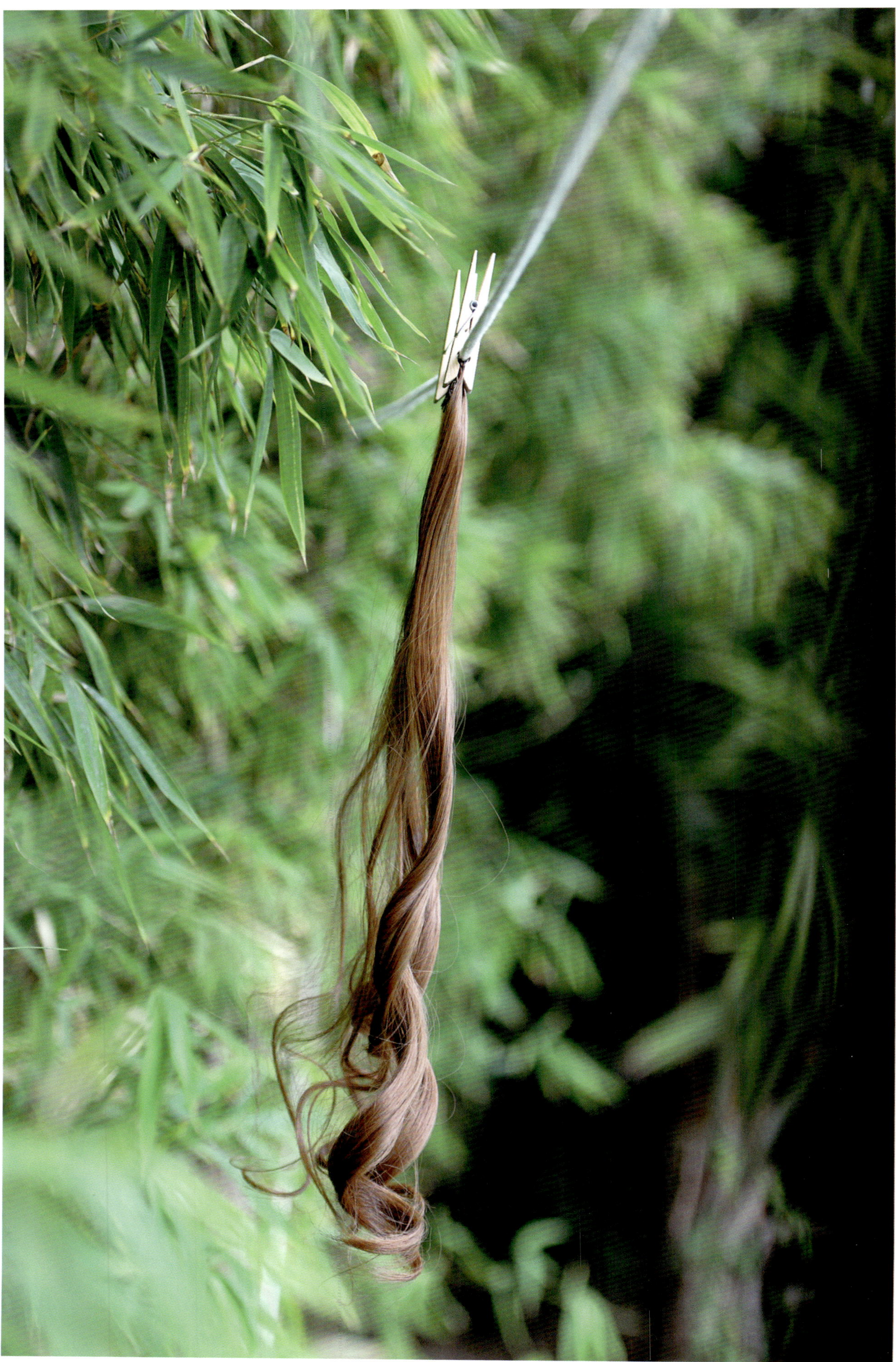

From an early age, I understood that hair had power. At the age of 7, my own two ponytails were chopped off very unceremoniously, and for a good part of my childhood, I sported a boy's haircut from which I probably never fully recovered. The trauma of losing control of my identity has stayed with me my entire life.

For my project *Hair Stories*, I interviewed and photographed almost three dozen women about their hair. These women represented a diverse group of ages (14 to 100) and ethnicities. The opening question was, "Tell me about your hair." What I discovered is that hair is a language, a shield, and a trophy Hair is a construct reflecting our identity, history, femininity, personality, our innermost feelings of self-doubt, aging, vanity, and self-esteem. Hair also has deep sociological roots. It can be indicative of a certain religious or political belief system and like its genetic code, is complicated and touches our very core.

The photographs in this series were inspired by the personal stories and histories of the subjects and created in their home environments. From my experience as a neurologist, I utilized the interviewing skills gleaned from medical training, and the women's oral narratives were transcribed and excerpted for written and audio clips.

Hair Stories reflects that hair is more than just style or aesthetics; it is a physical manifestation of the history of women. Every participant had her own unique connection to her hair (or the absence of it) and her own story, whether it was an association from childhood or a way of caring for or presenting her hair, yet there were many similarities in the language they used and the feelings expressed. The overall collective voice confirmed that hair is important and is best understood as a meaningful mirror of identity and often evolves, just as we do.

Rohina Hoffman

INTRODUCTION

In her first monograph, *Hair Stories*, photographer Rohina Hoffman uses her training and professional experience as a neurologist to explore the relationship that women have with their hair or lack thereof. The women she interviewed speak of rebirth, pride, coming of age, and of separation from institutionalized expectations. They also speak of fear, aging and death.

Hair can have the power to invigorate us and enhance our confidence, and adversely it can expose and alienate us. We make a statement with our hair.

There has been significant scholarship devoted to the history of hair throughout various cultures. You can find endless essays about the subject, and nowadays there are Instagram accounts devoted to the history and impact of hair. In a recent article in *The New York Times* entitled "Buzzed: The Politics of Hair," Vanessa Friedman explores the political power of women's hair as it relates to recent events, particularly in light of the #metoo movement. She focuses on what it means for a woman to make a political statement using hair as the mechanism. Does hair have that much influence?

The power of hair is certainly not only a women's issue, however it has long been associated with being female and is representative of the evolution of women throughout history. Short hair has come to symbolize defiance. Women shorn their hair as protesters, as martyrs, and as revolutionaries pushing against the status quo. In much of the West, short hair in the 1920s became associated with freedom, as women were simultaneously shaking loose the sartorial norms of the previous generations. Long hair takes time, care and money to upkeep. Short hair is liberating. Think of some well- known women such as Joan of Arc, Josephine Baker, Mia Farrow and Natalie Portman (to name a few) who made history not exclusively, but notably, because of their haircuts.

In the same Times article, Vanessa Friedman interviewed Princeton University lecturer Erin K. Vearncombe on the topic. Vearncome cites: "I don't think you can ever just shrug it [hair] off as a matter of personal expression," she says, "Hair is intrinsically linked to assumptions about gender and power relations." [Vanessa Friedman, "Buzzed: The Politics of Hair," *The New York Times*, April 5, 2018.].

Long hair has undoubtedly been aligned with femininity, health and fertility. Long hair represents youth. In Ancient Roman and Greek cultures, women's long hair became a symbol of sexuality and abundance. Today it is still seen by men and women as a sign of sexual, feminine identity.

Modern women have been taught to attend to our hair from a young age. Consider the plethora of cultural references about women's hair in films, television, music and social media. The impact is significant. Hair remains a topic often overlooked and yet integral to how we define ourselves. *Hair Stories* is evidence of this.

Upon first glance, the photographs in *Hair Stories* intrigue and invite us to learn about the subjects captured. The images require the accompanying text, and the text naturally relies upon the photographs. However, it is worth examining Hoffman's images of her subjects with care and without the text. Taking in each image for a few moments allows us to become captivated by the subject. It is valuable to remember that photographs tell numerous stories. We can learn a lot about both the photographer and the subject from a photograph, in the choices both make in taking and posing. In many cases, our assumptions about a picture create new, fictionalized stories about the subject and what they represent to us. That is the magic and complexity inherent in photography.

To look at Hoffman's photographs is to understand strangers through her lens. Some of her pictures depict women in motion: dancing, swaying, jumping. Other pictures depict texture, vibrant color, and theatrics. Hoffman chose to photograph her subjects in their homes, rather than in a studio, allowing for a more intimate and authentic setting. The powerful images in the book reveal something about the subject beyond their hair: their pain, loss, spirit. There is explicit happiness and sadness in the photographs, and the artist captures both successfully. In a few stories, women discuss using their hair as a protective mechanism against society, or against their fears. A woman reflects on losing her hair, and the liberation she finds as a result. For some women, spending effort on their hair is an extension of self-care; for others, leaving their hair in its natural state is a symbol of freedom. Hair acts as a cloak, it physically shields the face. We may not be able to see someone's eyes or expression when their hair is in the way. Hair can also expose a person, and humble them. Hair becomes a symbol of our spirit.

In Hoffman's *Hair Stories*, we come to understand strangers through the experience of transformation. The photographs and text offer us subtle and profound lessons about these strangers, and we learn about them in a way that is accessible to all of us. Hair provides the artist and her subjects with a platform for connection and we as viewers are left with greater compassion and understanding of others.

Emily Lambert-Clements
Art Advisor & Former Associate Director at Fraenkel Gallery, S.F.

BRUSHED OFF: ON WHY HAIR MATTERS

My mother died of cancer in 2015.

She had bright red hair, the kind that lights up in the sun.

I was with her when the hairdresser shaved it off, anticipating the ravages of chemotherapy. I gathered it up, saving her hair as a lifeline to what I once knew, and keep it in a small box.

My mother's hair is still radiant, glossy, and lifelike. It is too saturated with emotion, too charged with her essence, to ever be thrown away.

Public and malleable, our hair defines our identity. When severed and saved after death, it keeps memory alive, preserving a physical connection to our ancestors. Hair is alive and immortal, not only because it does not age, but also because of the talismanic power we invest in it.

Yet hair is frequently trivialized as a lifeless body part or frivolous beauty accessory. It is devalued as both the object of vanity and subject of mundane bodily practices like washing, brushing, primping, and pruning.

In fact, hair is ambiguous. It is made up of dead skin cells that grow from a scalp alive with blood vessels and bacterial life. It splits, sheds, and re-grows, acting as the body's renewable resource. And although it exists as dead matter on the margins of clinical medicine, its vitality is often valued in medical discussion as the gauge of a healthy body.

Similarly, in commodity culture, ample hair growth is a sign of vibrant and "successful" femininity—a measure infused by Western ideologies of mainstream beauty, rooted in the dogma of Biblical times. "Long hair" is, as St. Paul assures us, a woman's crowning "glory," but must be covered for the vanity it displays and the lust it inspires in men (1 Corinthians 11:15).

Being without hair can be emotional and depersonalizing. Forced haircuts and head shaving are among the many dehumanizing measures aimed at torturing and humiliating prisoners, from Auschwitz to Abu Ghraib. Additionally, in a rare exposé in the *New Zealand Herald* entitled "Black Gold," which investigates China's lucrative commercial hair supply, girls who sell their braids weep when the haircuts are complete, presumably feeling diminished.

If hair forms such a vibrant part of who we are, and how we stay connected to others, why is it routinely underestimated as a serious subject matter?

This question is imbued with political dimensions, for what makes something matter—or not matter—is the product of human decision, with those in power determining who and what counts as they write history. French historian and philosopher Michel Foucault (1976) suggests power produces (and reproduces) knowledge by shaping it to serve its own interests, as in the patriarchal determination to subdue women and devalue femininity.

Our culture aligns the feminine with frivolity and a lack of substance and pairs the masculine with gravity. The feminization and subsequent trivializing of hair is intellectually rooted in classical antiquity and Christianity, but became especially salient with the onset of European capitalist modernity in the late eighteenth and nineteenth centuries, when men's hairstyles became shorter and less elaborate.

What resulted was a Western fascination with women's hair: think of Dante Gabriel Rossetti's flame-haired Pre-Raphaelite muses, or John Milton's disheveled Eve in *Paradise Lost*, popularly depicted in nineteenth-century illustration. However, the ample depictions of women's hair were not just aesthetic. They also communicated the social and moral position of women in the eyes of men.

Layered into women's hair stories were populist framings of self-indulgence and unproductive materialism. Hair worship became synonymous with women's trivial interests: too personal, physical, and vapid to be of any significance.

The inherent critique of women's bodies and alleged vanity implies women cannot be trusted with authority or power, a legacy that survives today. Recall the lead-up to the 2016 US presidential election, when internet trolls used Hillary Clinton's changing hairstyles as evidence of her incompetence.

The benefit of such an example is, as feminist author Laurie Penny writes on hair, it "make[s] misogyny legible." That is, it shows how hair/styling has been used to give material form to mechanisms of power and control like sexism, racism, and colonialism.

In the building of America, for example, slavers, explorers, and "scientists" classified African hair textures as ugly and animal-like, justifying subjugation, enslavement, and death. But just as hair has been a place for domination to manifest and multiply, so too have its strands and styles been sites for resistance to play out. Consider that, in colonial Colombia, African slaves plaited secret messages and escape routes into women's hair, facilitating freedom through the language of braid patterns.

Today, we see political resistance in women's collective and individual actions: from the natural hair movement, or the acceptance of hair loss, to the pleasure derived from a great hairdo or fabulous wig. Hair stories, (as this book is titled), become lifelines to a more intimate understanding of our lives, our culture, our histories, our politics, and ourselves, especially in the face of grief, pain, and loss.

Through candid portraits of a diverse group of women interviewed about their hair, Rohina Hoffman exposes the personal, emotional, and political significance our tresses carry. In light of recent social change, and the broadening of feminist perspectives in the age of Trump, the importance of Hoffman's *Hair Stories* is clear.

By giving a voice to women, and highlighting women's agency and power through their most potent emblem, this project challenges the ideologies that support the subordination of women, and that diminish the feminine. Far from secondary, superfluous, or spiritless, as *Hair Stories* shows, hair is central in the lives of women and vital to human understanding.

Esther R. Berry
Fashion and gender studies scholar and curator
Ryerson University, Toronto

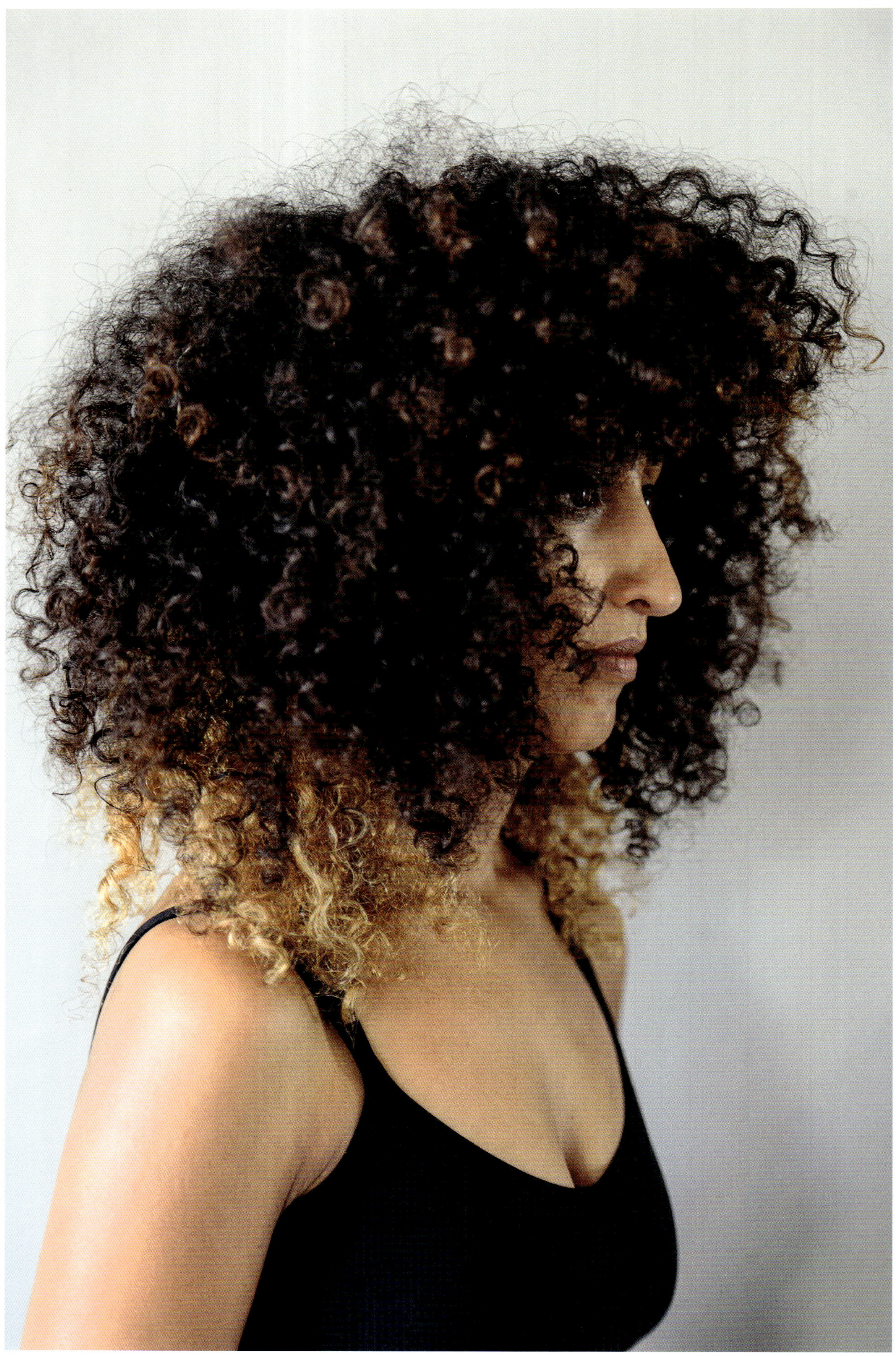

yasmine

When I was 19, two of my sisters and I cut ties with our family. I had someone I was supposed to marry and I wasn't going to do that. Within a year of leaving I started wearing my hair naturally. It took me years to figure out what to do with it, and how to handle it, because it was like a rebirth. I was finally free.

As girls, we were not allowed to cut it, as we grew up in a patriarchal community and family. Gender roles were very clear-cut and there was no ambiguity. I didn't realize how much broader society affected the way I saw my hair. Everyone I idolized in pop culture had "nice" straight hair. (Afros weren't in when I was growing up and didn't seem cool to me.)

Nineteen years later, I had a Skype call with my mother for the first time, and my hair was up in a bun. "Let me see your hair," she said. So I took out the hair tie, and the first thing she said was, "You like it like that?"

Clearly after a 19 year absence, there were a lot more important things to talk about than the state of my hair!

With dreads, it's like, when they grow out, a part of your soul is growing into them. So it's not just how you're presenting yourself. It's not just influencing you and your personality. It's literally a part of you. It's like you are putting your soul into that hair.

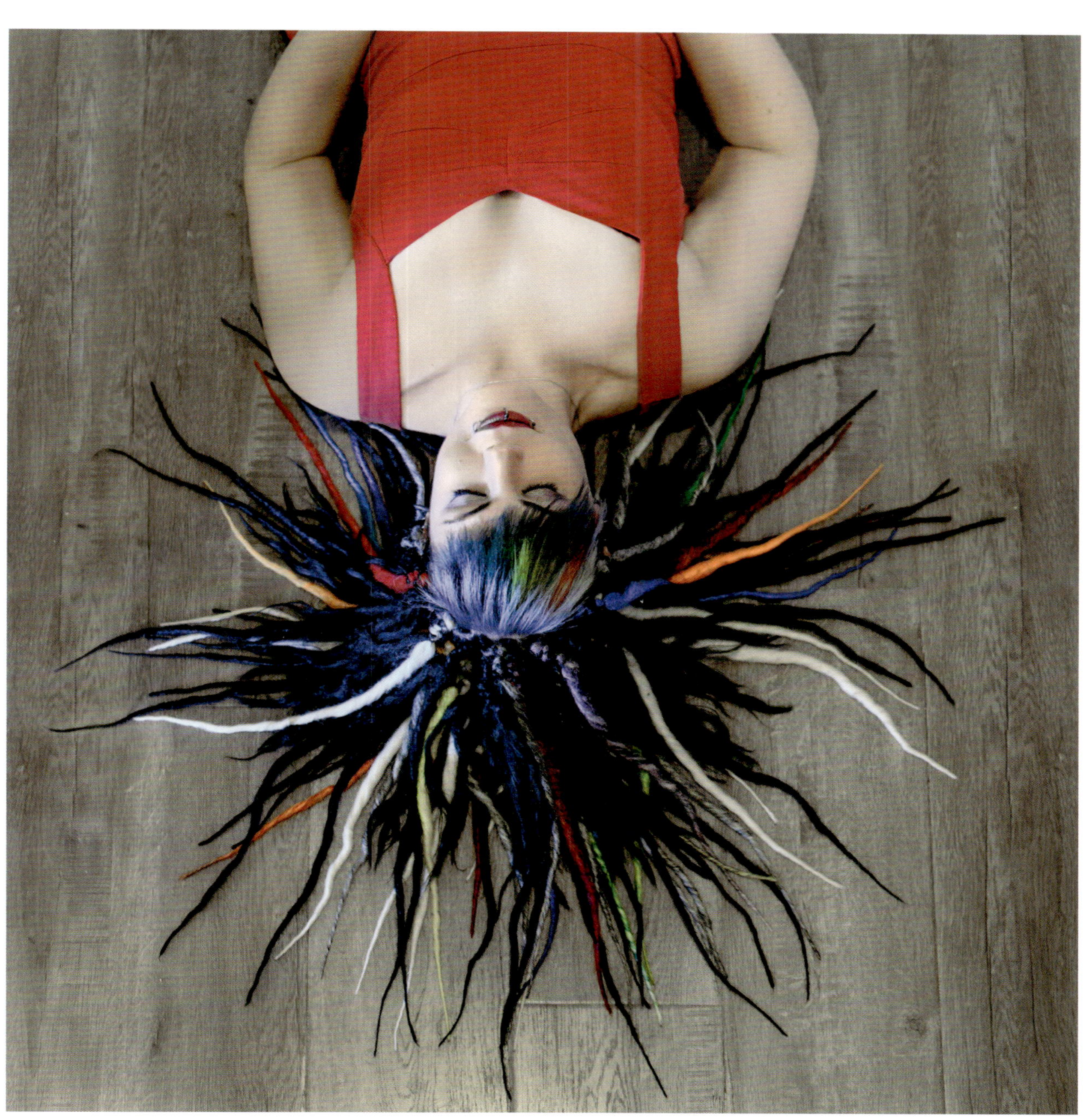

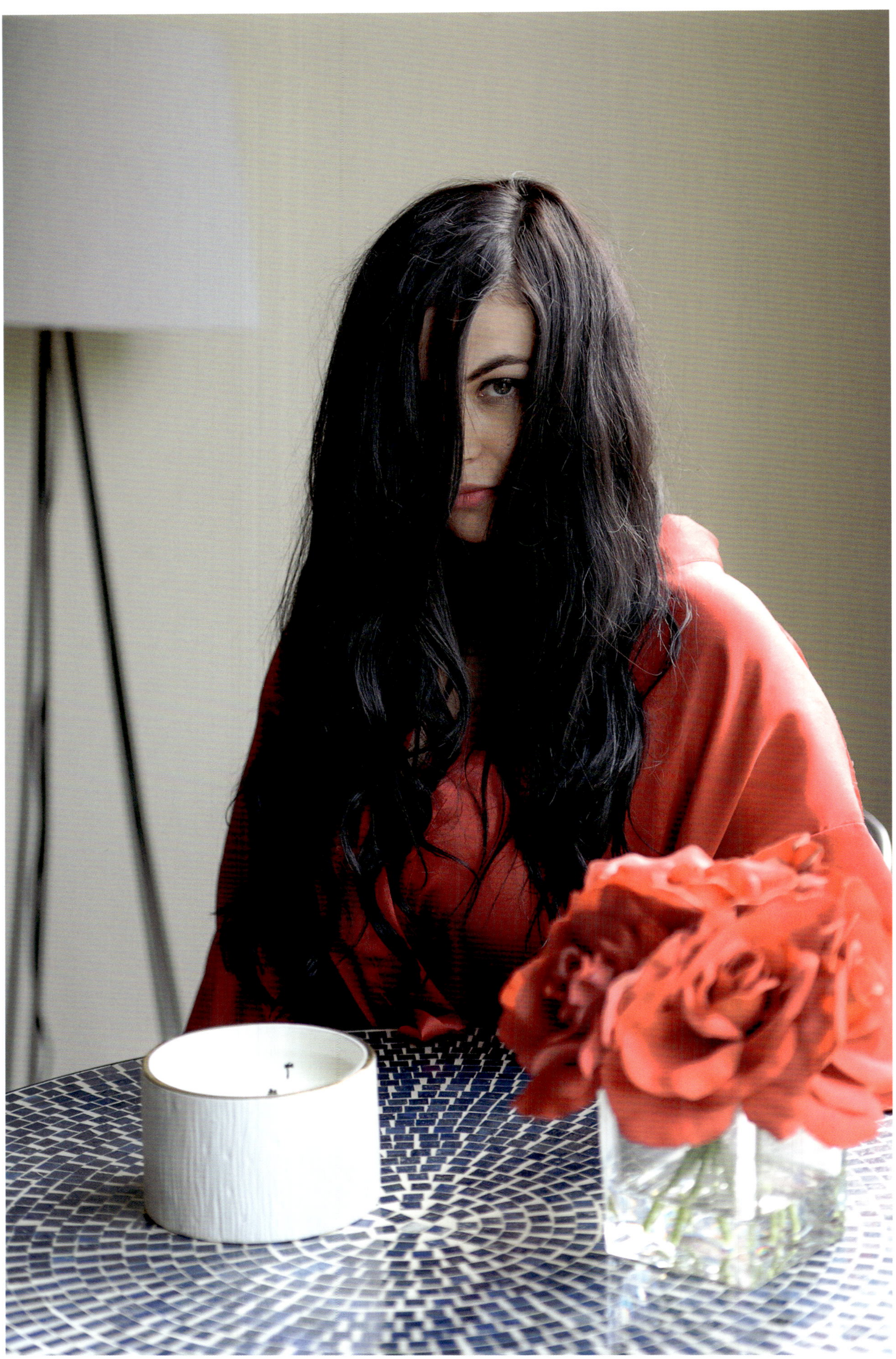

larisa

When I was in first grade, my mom took me to the salon and cut my hair really short like a boy. She thought it was adorable. I cried for days. Ever since, I've had long hair. It took years to grow out, and it takes a lot for me to get haircuts. I don't get more than an inch cut off at a time.

Long hair makes me feel more feminine, and my entire style is geared towards that. I can't see myself cutting it short.

sophie

In middle school, I tried really hard to suppress my hair's natural texture and make it straight like everyone else's. All I wanted was really long, straight, blond hair. It's been three months since I decided to let my hair do its own thing. Go natural. And it's funny, because a lot of my friends who have curly hair are doing the exact same thing. We've all ditched the flat-irons and blow-dryers and are just wearing our hair natural.

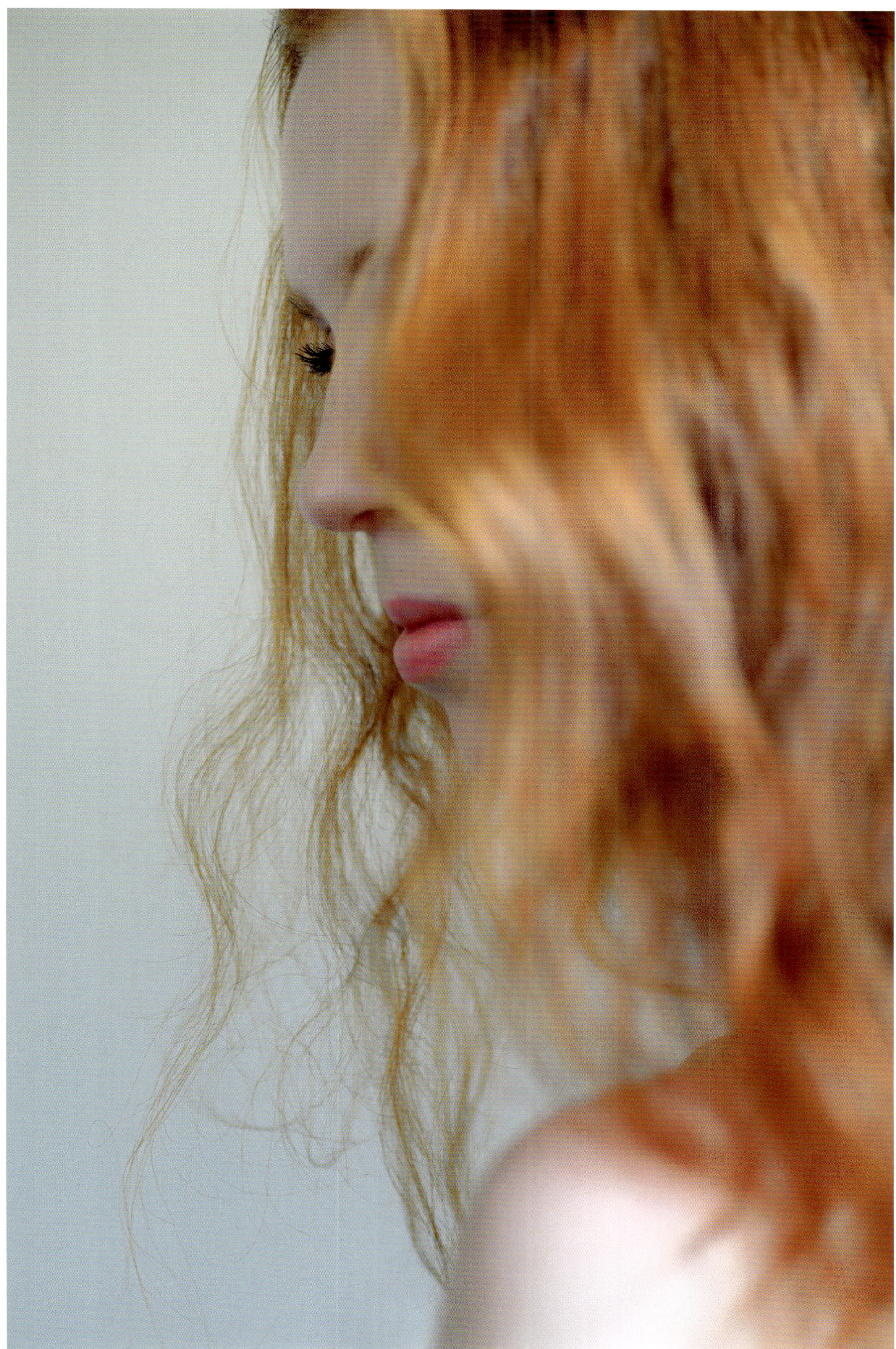

susan

I just finished chemo, so I'll see what happens. I never chose to wear a wig because this is me. I'm not trying to hide myself from anyone. If I don't have any hair, I'm not going to put something false on my head, as I wouldn't inject my lips or do Botox. (It's an "I'm as old as I am kind of thing.") I've met so many women who stop me and ask questions and share their stories.

Sometimes, they just hold my arm for a moment. I never mind.

To cross the chasm is magical.

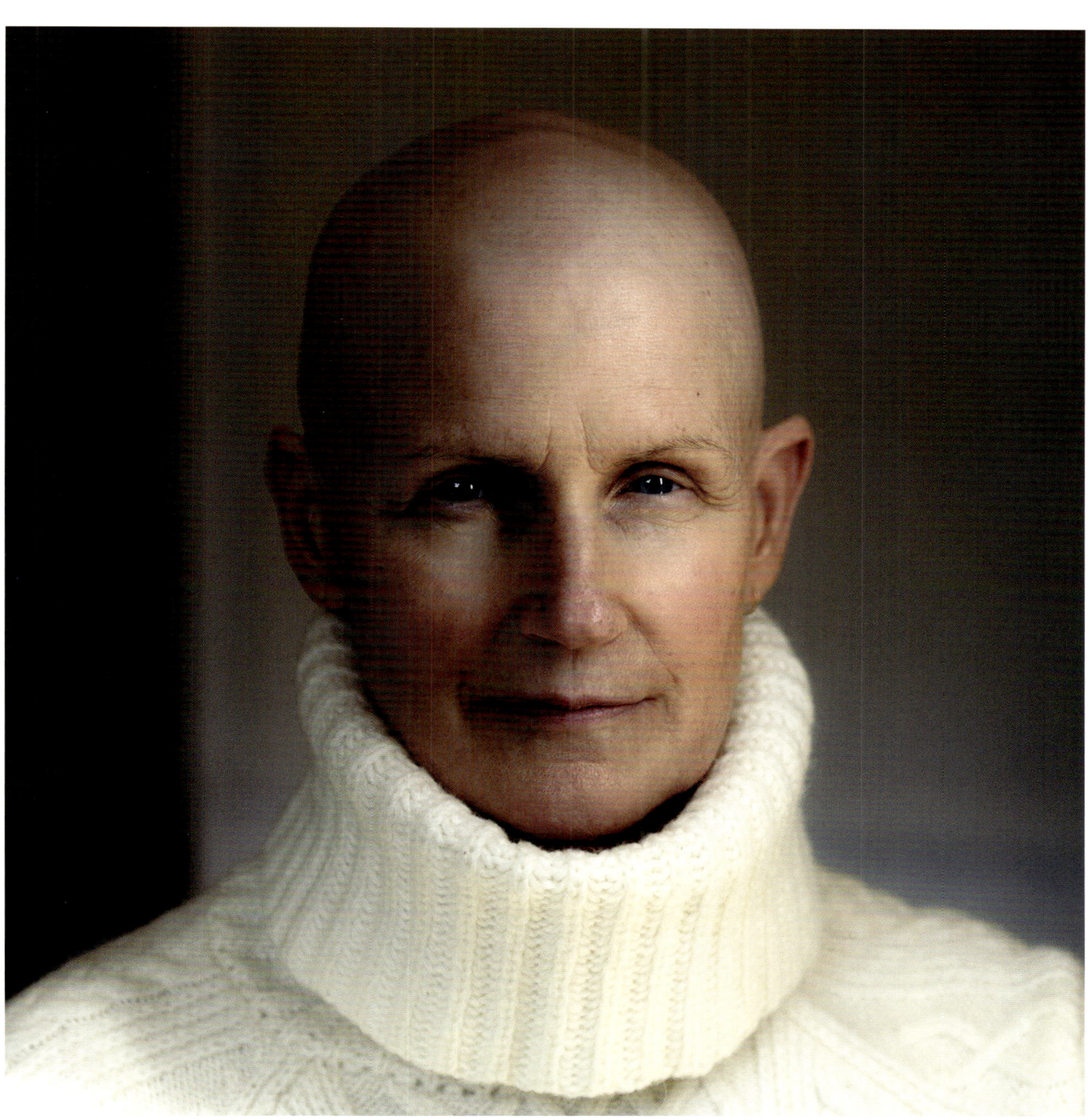

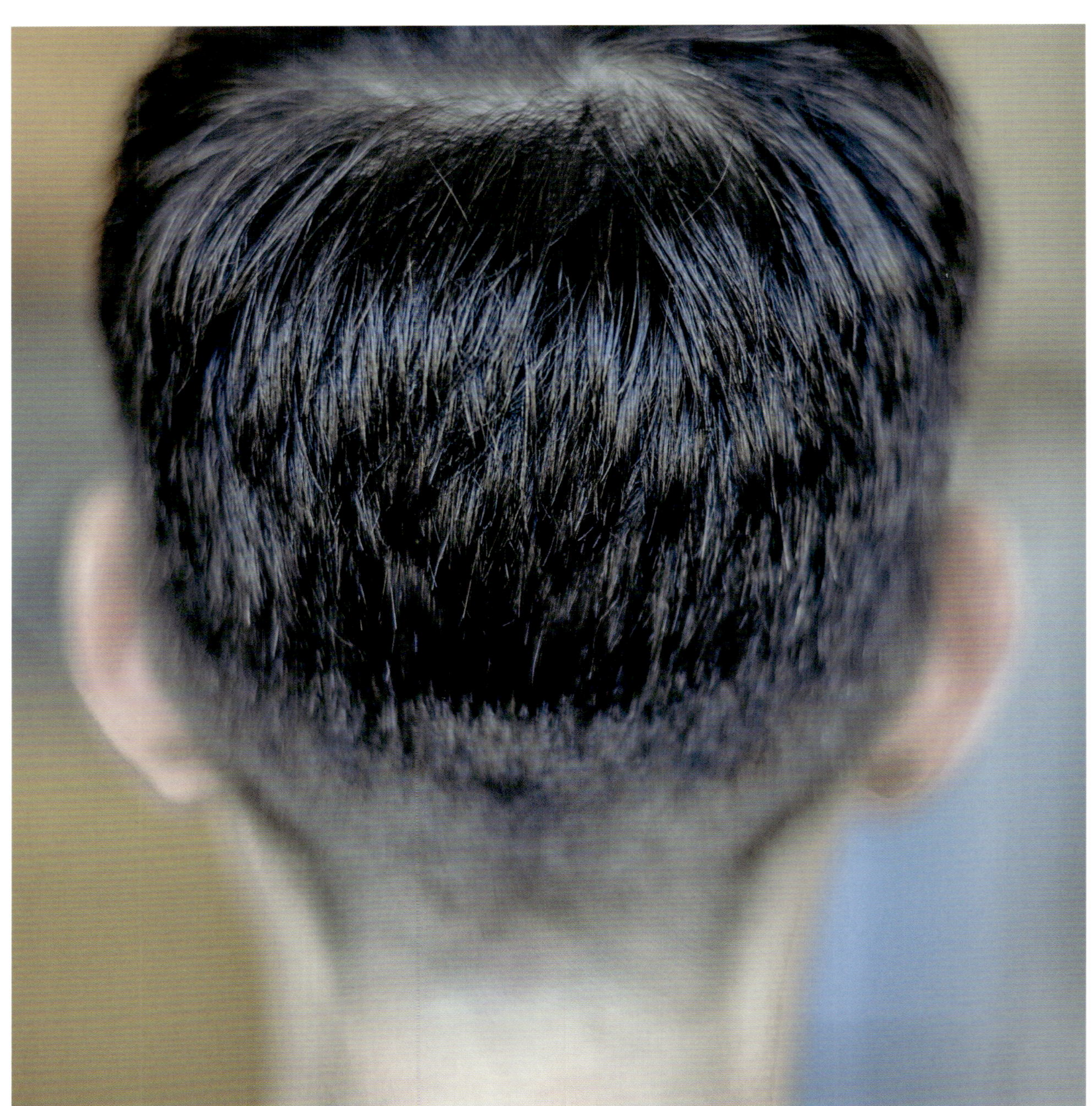

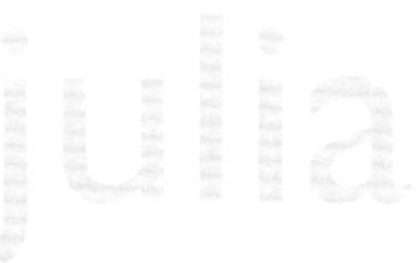

I was always asked a lot as a kid, "Why do you want to be a boy?" I never understood that because I didn't want to be a boy. I was very happy being a girl but I wanted to be a tomboy. I didn't even like the word tomboy. I wanted to be a tomgirl, or a Jane of all trades, or a Julia of all trades.

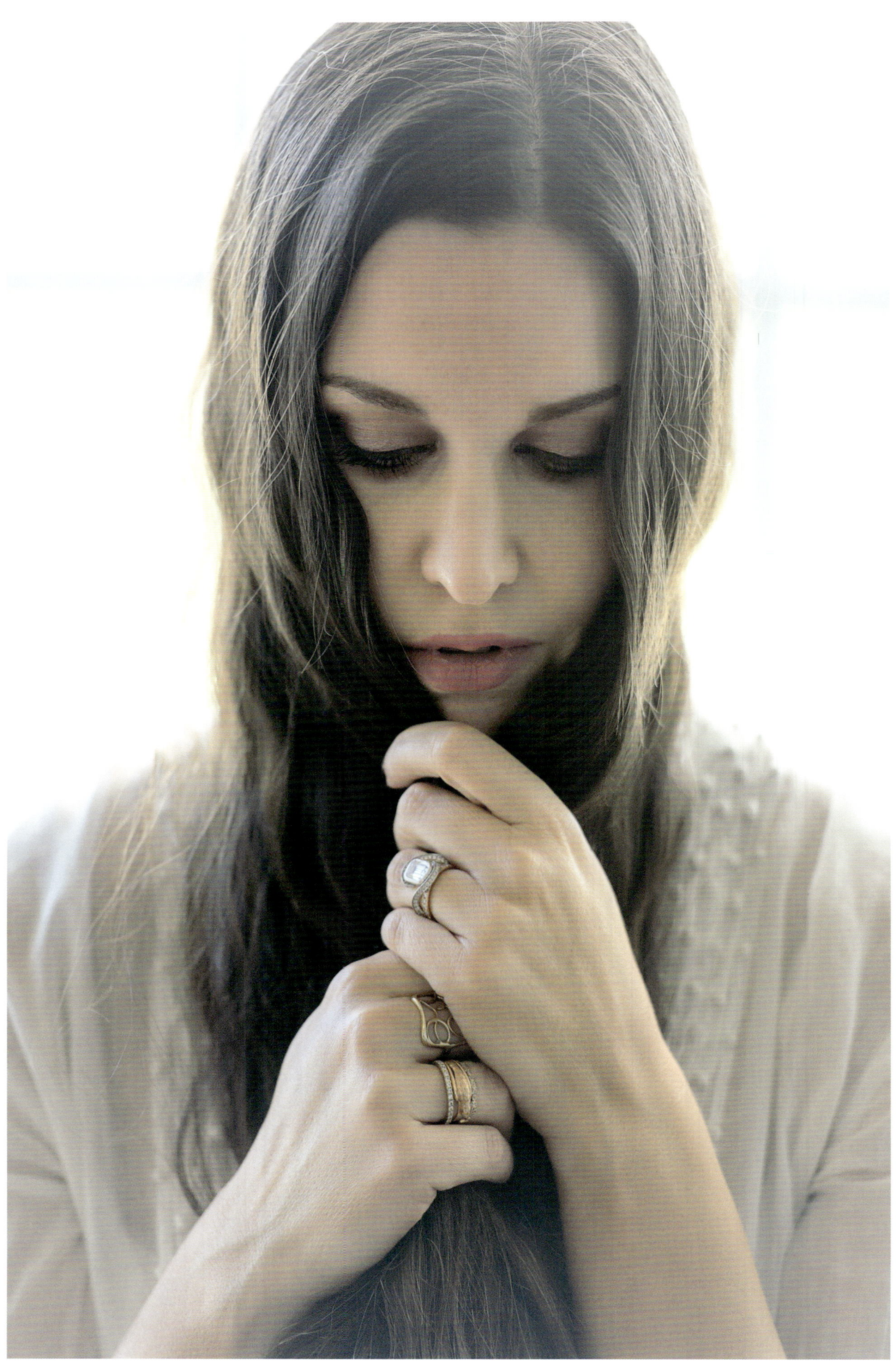

alexis

I have all of this hair and I can hide behind it. I am a mother of three children; happy but tired. If I didn't hide, you'd see a scared woman, unsure about the future. Where is my place in things? I'm so happy I have a wonderful husband and three children, but I still think there is more, though I'm not sure what it is yet.

barbara

I've had the same hairdresser since my 40s.

I go to the beauty parlor once a week to see him. He's very definite on what he likes and thinks a certain look is for me. He's a hard person to argue with because he's very definite in his opinions. Sometimes, I'd like to try something else, but I'm nervous about switching. He just will not budge on his styling.

He would say, "I want to try this. I want to make your hair a bit longer on top." I think it's okay and really don't like it after he's done, but I just put up with it because he's so strong-minded. I'm a little nervous to say, "I don't like that. I want to go back to the other one." I'm kind of worried he might say, "No, this is better for you."

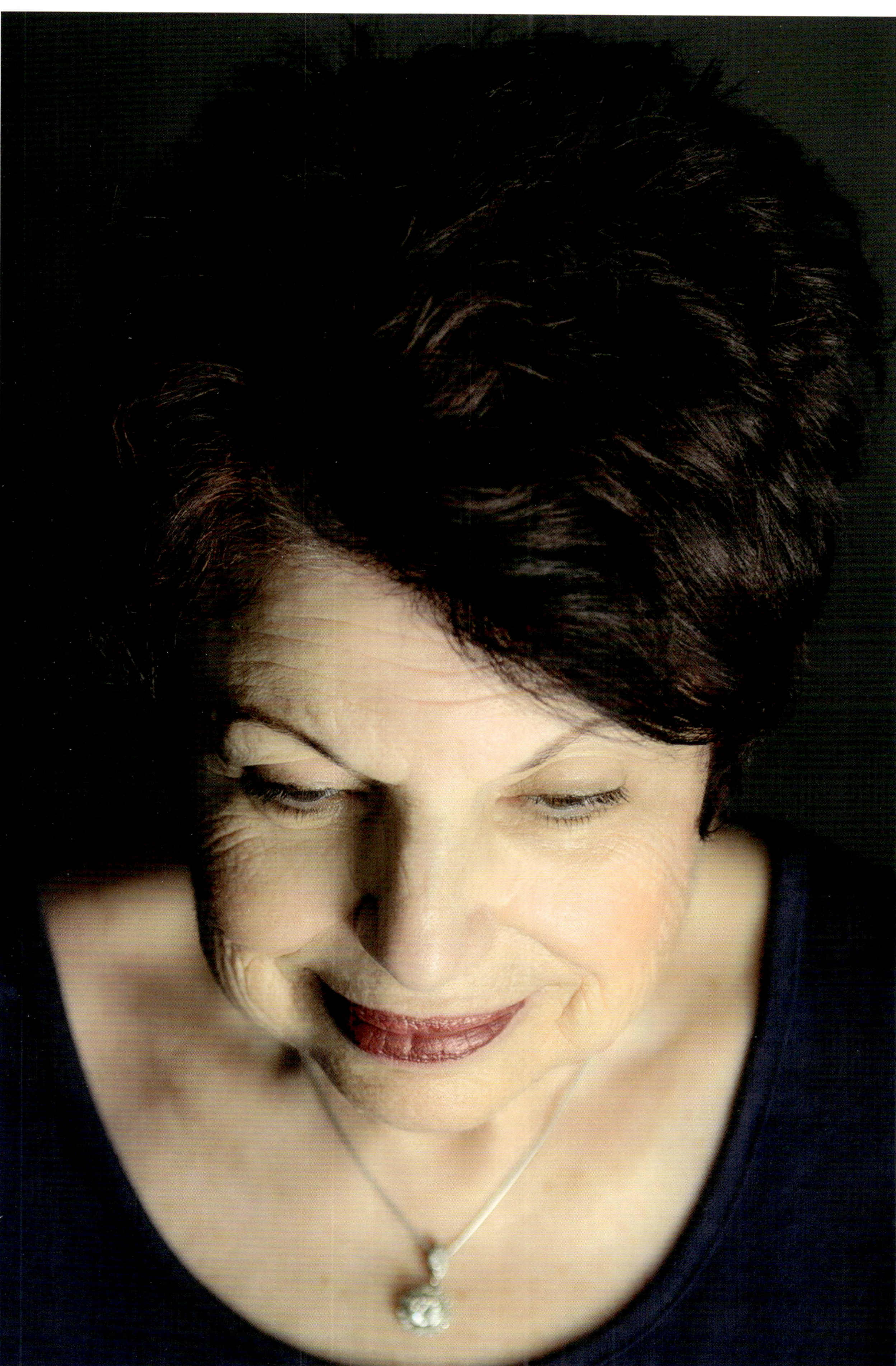

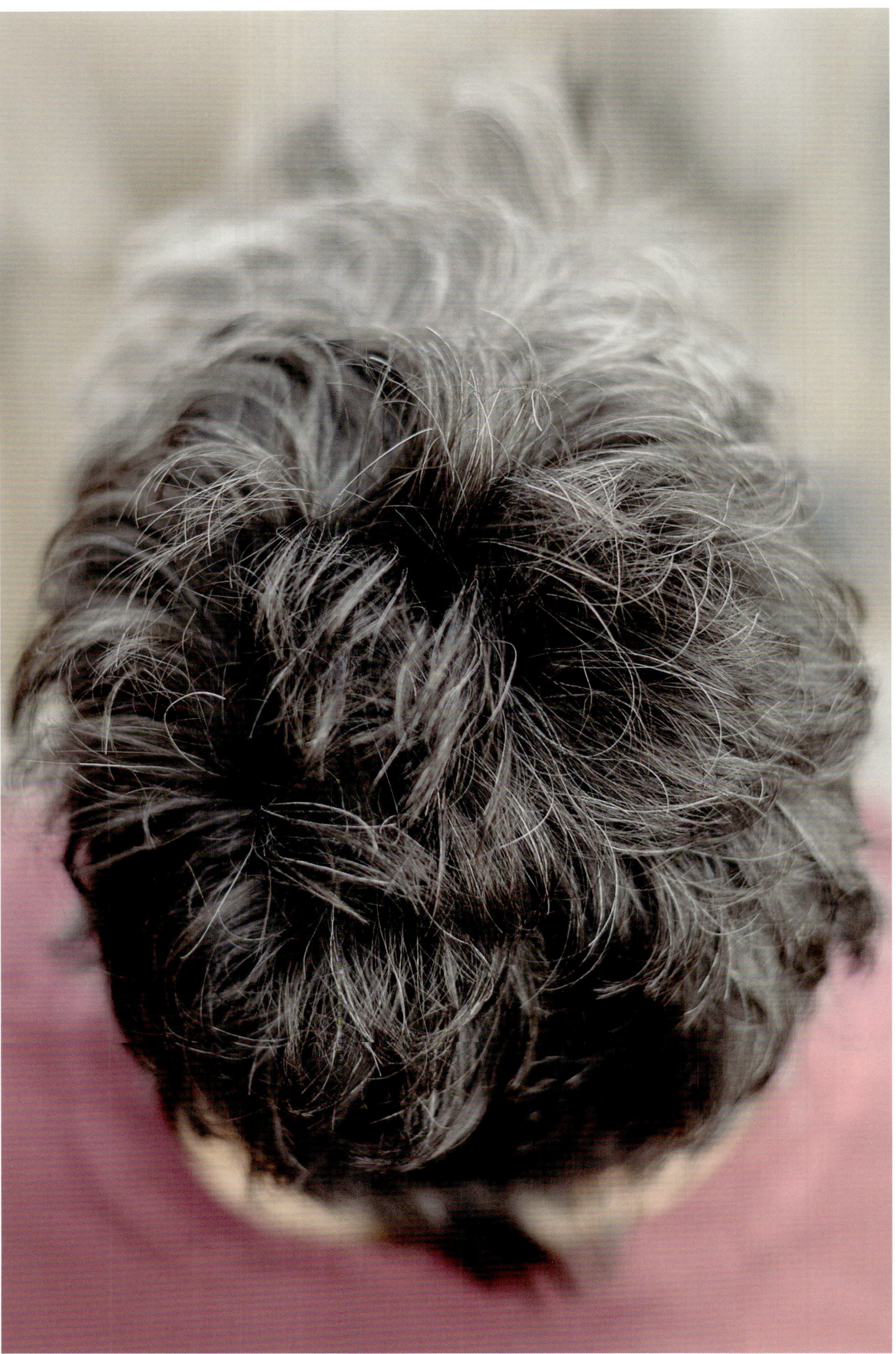

My hair first went gray in my 50s. I actually want more gray.

It's coming in very slowly. I liked the contrast, and it didn't really phase me. It's coming in silver but I would like more! I have this friend, and it looks like she has a light behind her. That's how it glows, her hair. I would like that glow. It's a cool thing. I know young people are actually dying their hair gray.

marissa

My hair is everything and rules my life.

If I'm having a bad day, and I go for a blow-dry, everything is so much better. I've been doing weekly blow-drys for seven years, at least. I never buy shampoo or conditioner because I haven't washed my own hair in seven years.

Water cannot get near my hair. (I'm like a gremlin.) I always carry a hat, hood, and an umbrella with me, and when rain is involved, it's a big deal. I turn into that scary woman that needs to grab a newspaper, a bag, or whatever is there, and put it over her head.

Do not let any water on my hair.

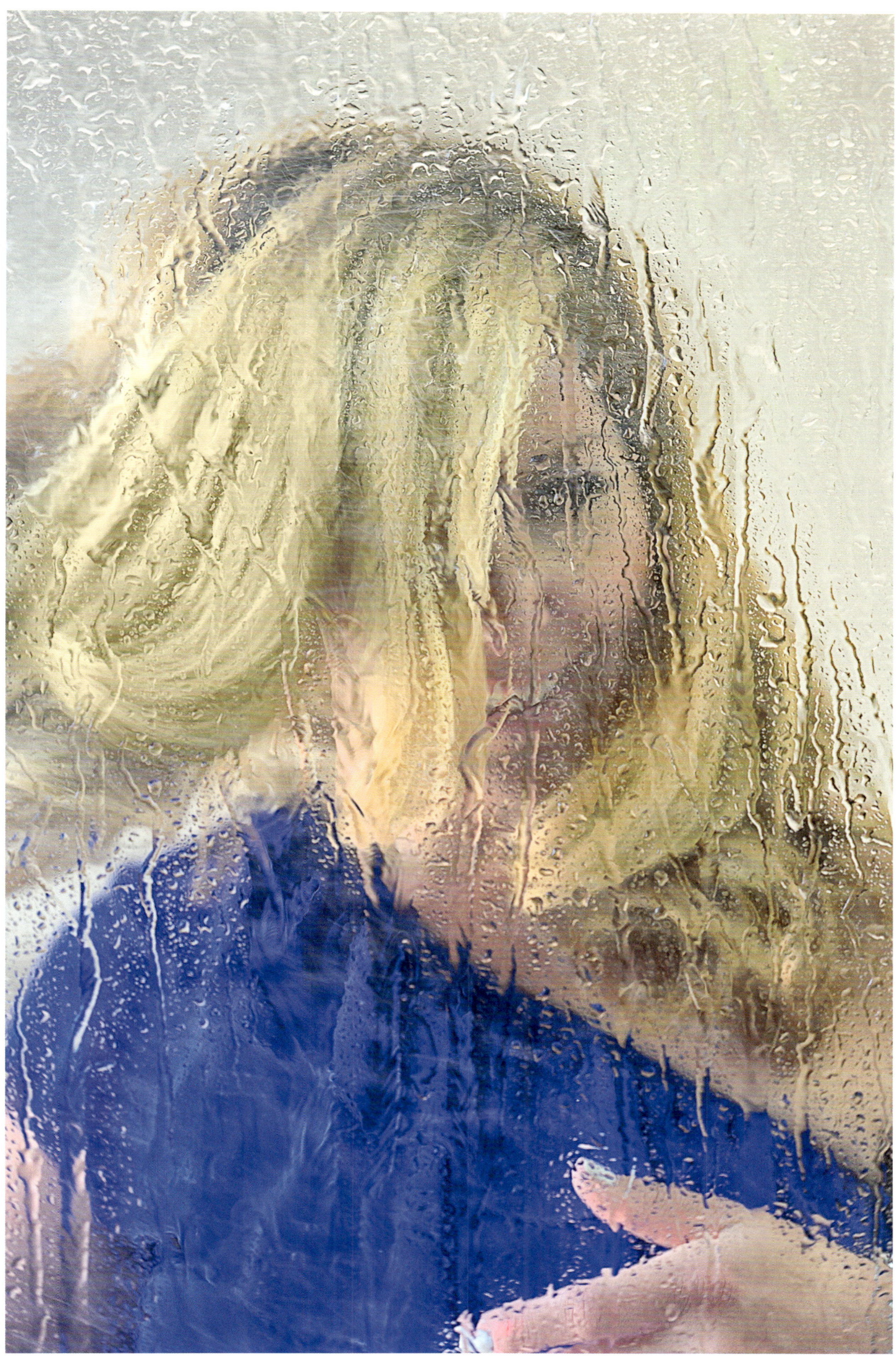

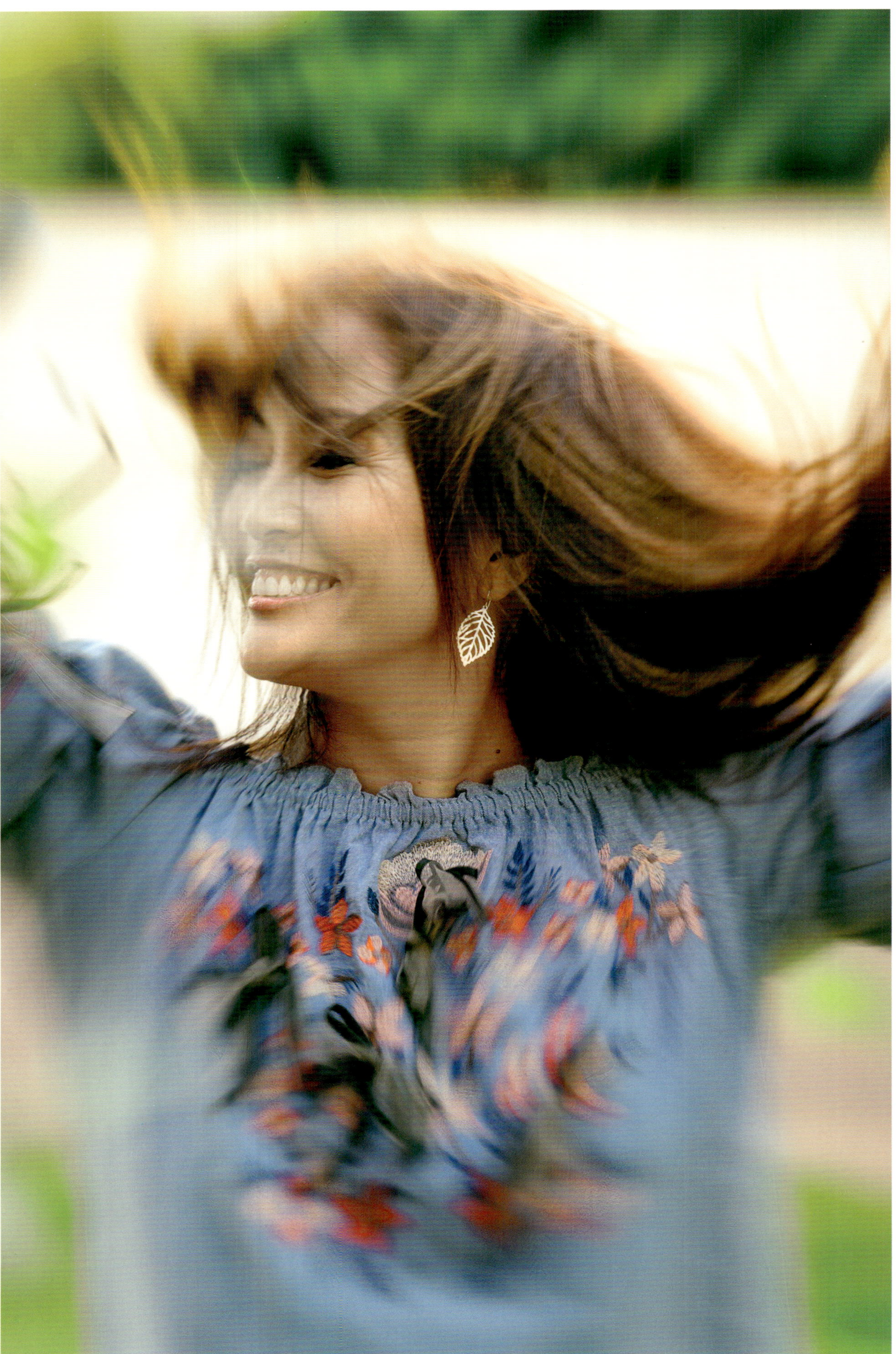

carrie ann

I have very specific ideas about how to do my hair because it's an important part of the way I feel when I walk out onto set.

On the TV show "Dancing with the Stars," where I'm a judge, usually around Week 5, the contestants start to get more uncomfortable with our comments (if they're not doing well.) They're feeling hurt and I'm sensitive to that.

I'll make sure to soften my hair so what I say comes off softer. If I do it in a severe style every word I say will come across like an ice pick. If there's a time when I feel I need to be tougher then I come in with slightly straighter hair.

Stick-straight.

brooke

With Miss America, hair was part of my costume, a part of my brand, "What does my hair say about me?"

I remember thinking, "Okay, I'm going to wear my hair the same in every area of competition: evening gown, talent, and interview. Every time they see me, they'll remember that one thing about me."

I've tried all kinds of different things including blonde extensions. I guess my complex was that my hair was never big enough. It was always really thin, and kind of flat and I always wanted more body. I wanted it bigger and louder.

I feel like I spend all of my time trying to plump my hair.

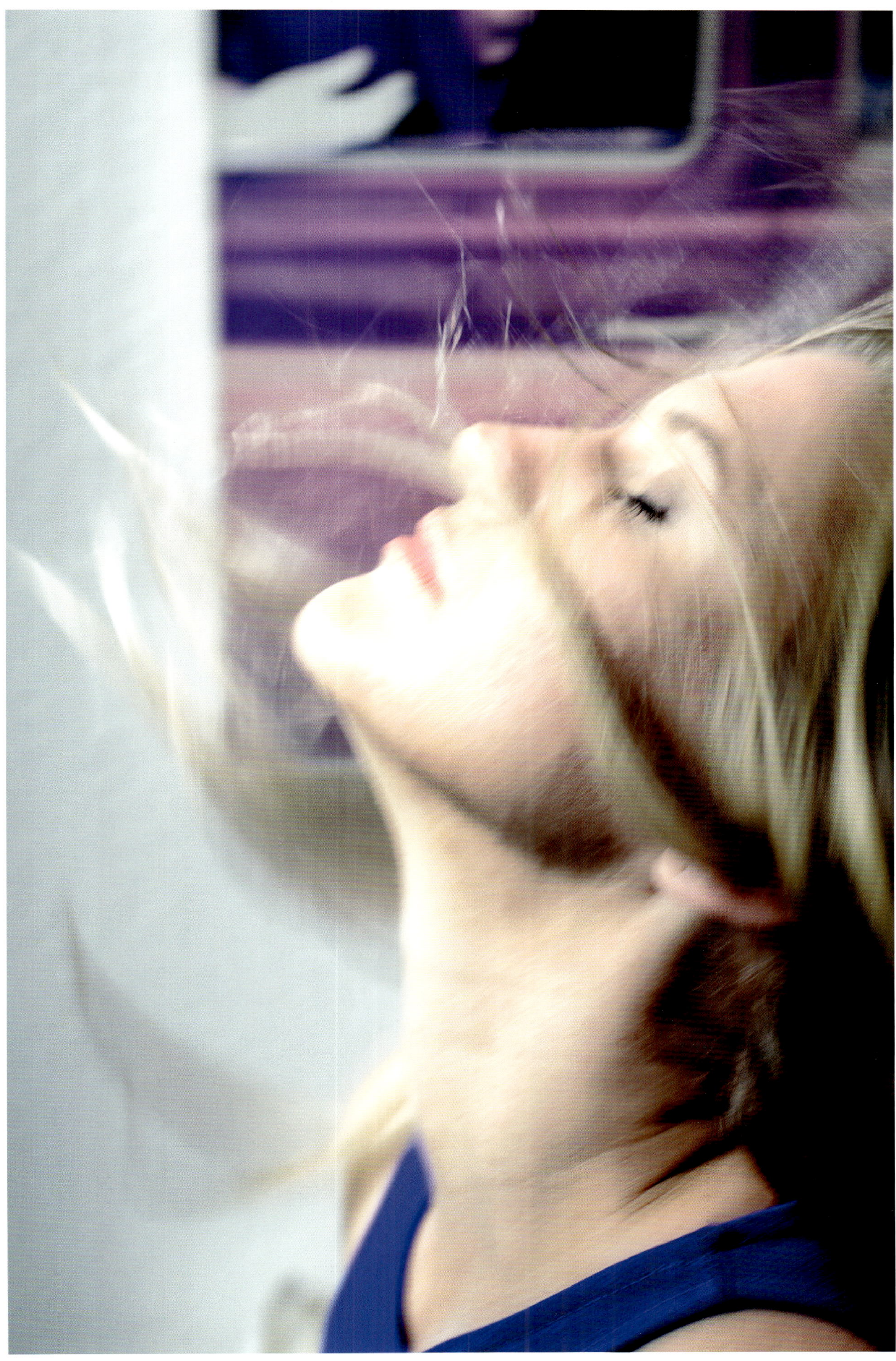

ogy

My mother is Algerian, and my dad is Black, American-Indian, and Irish. I was born with a full head of black curly hair.

There was nobody that looked like me, nobody that had hair like mine, and nobody that could tell me what the heck to use. I had this alien stuff on my head that nobody knew what to do with, and it was up to me to figure it out.

I meet a boy. We start dating; we break up. I have a revelation that it was my hair. That's the reason why we broke up, because my hair wasn't good enough.

There's this drive of, "If I fix my hair, everything in the world will be fine. My world will be fine. It'll be in control." It's so important to see ourselves reflected back being told, "This is beautiful. This is good too."

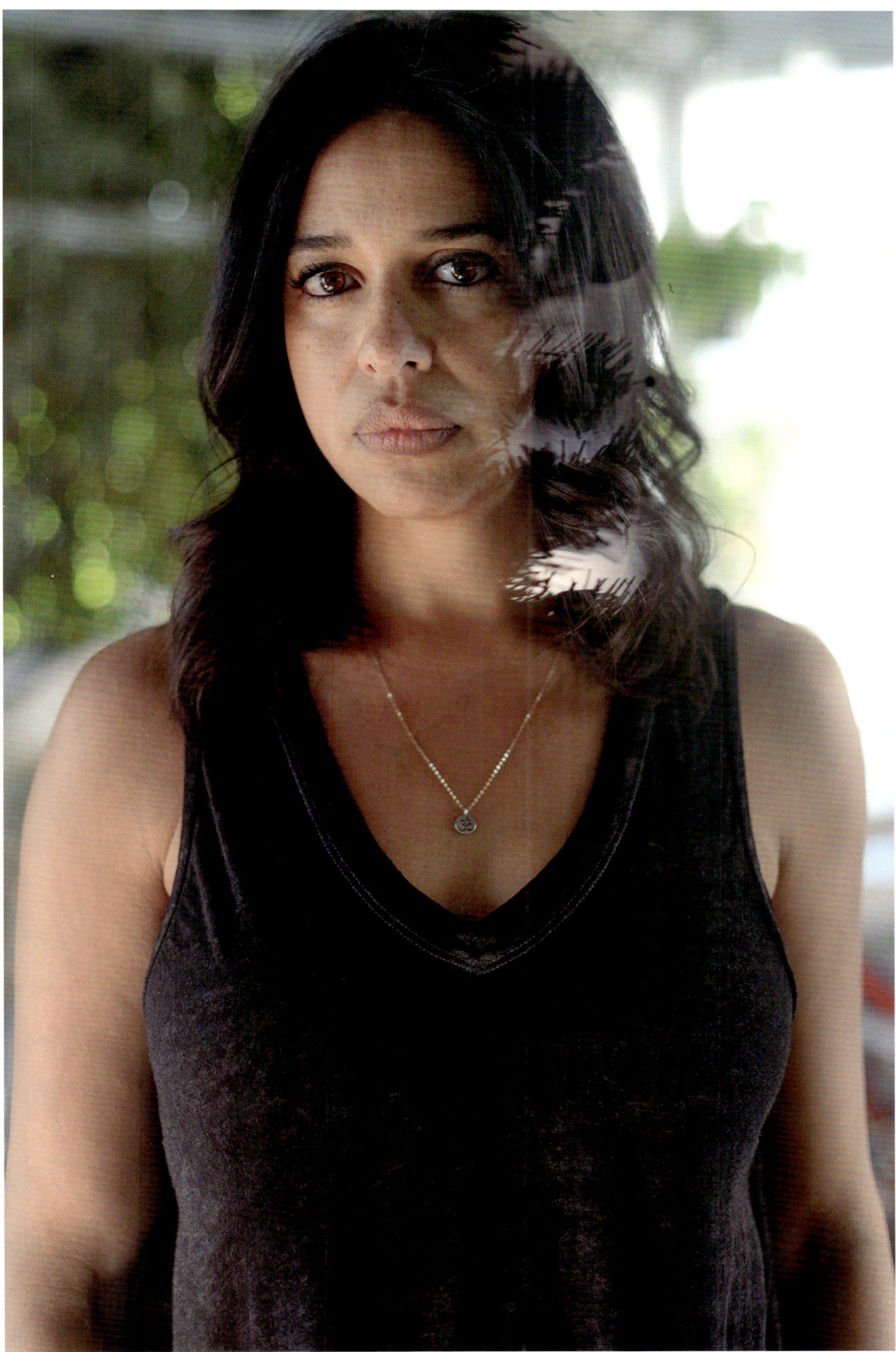

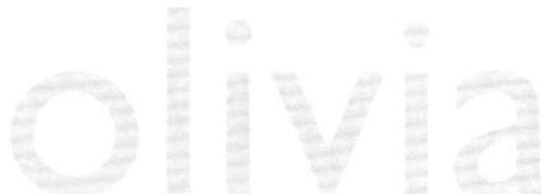

I love my hair. It's always been long. People always comment on it and want to touch it. I've never colored it. I like natural everything. I don't wear much makeup and don't paint my nails. I'm happy with myself.

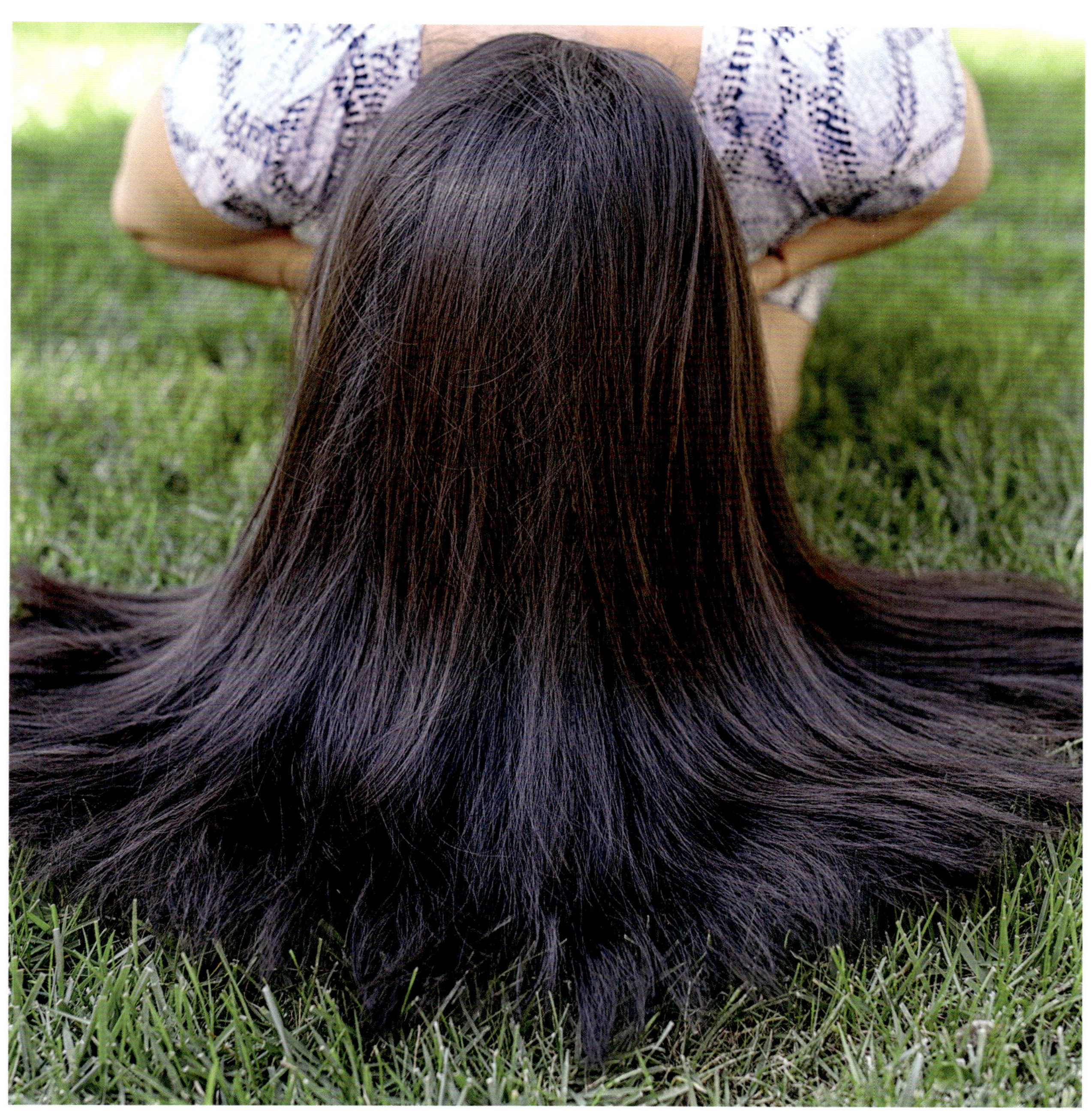

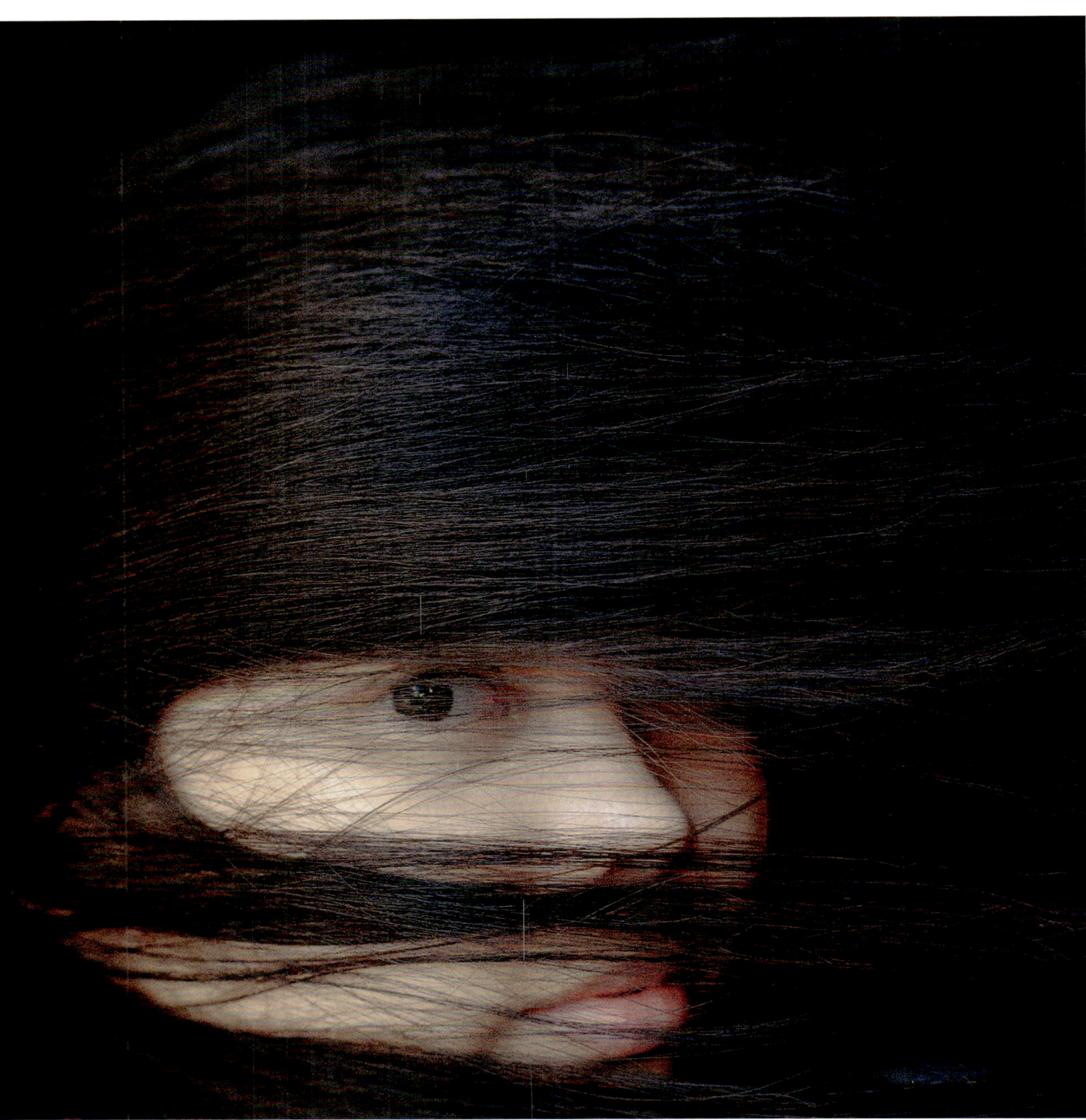

althea

I think I will always have long hair. It is kind of like my shield. It's a cover up from being judged by others.

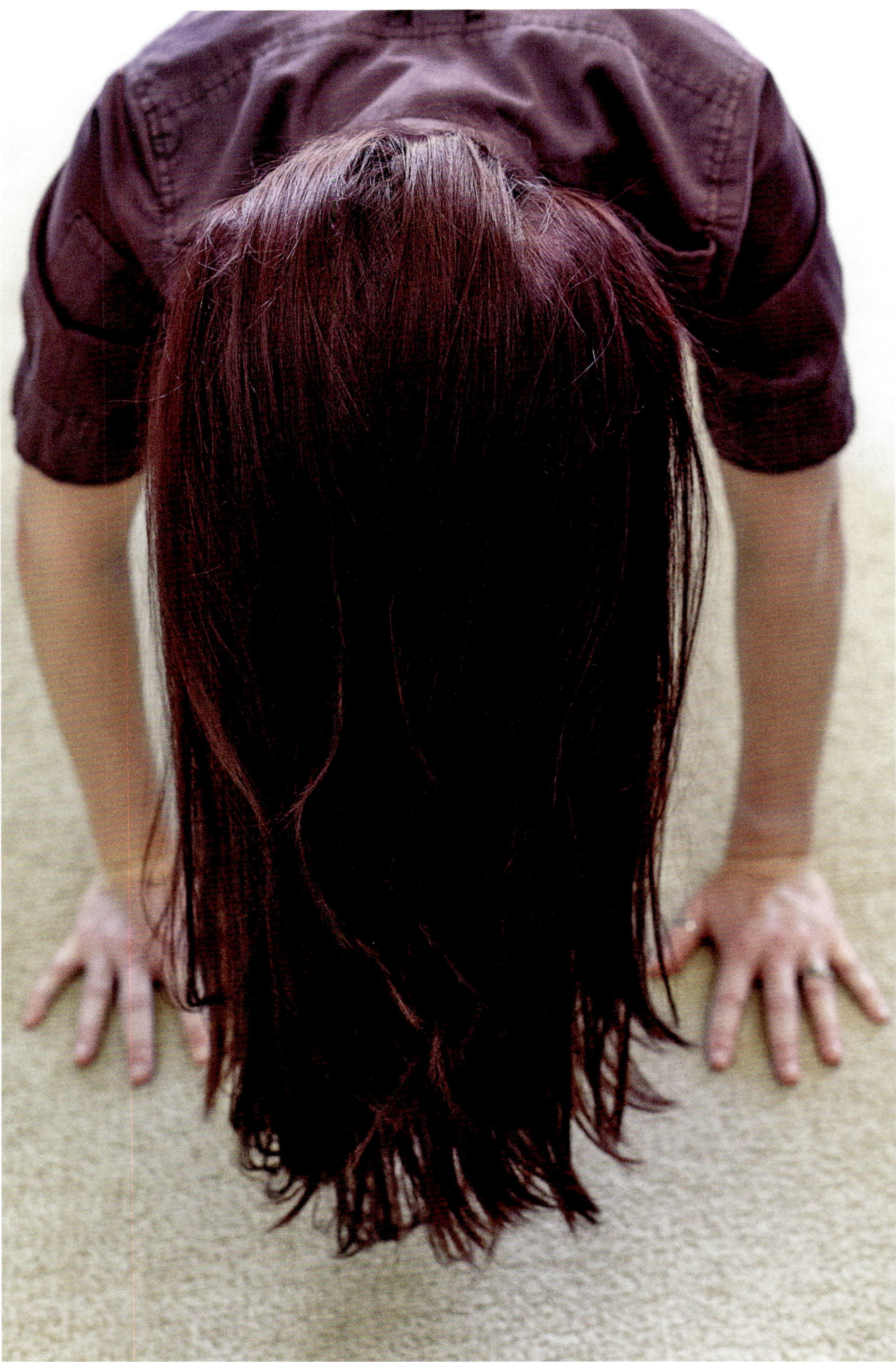

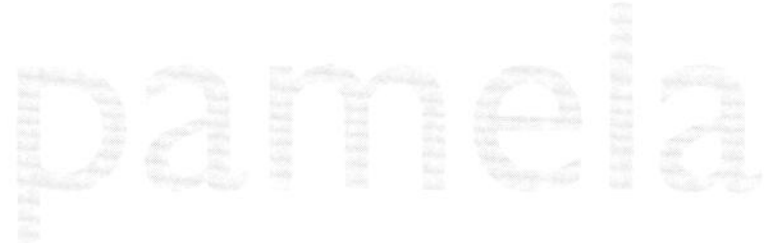

I was born a blonde but I dye my hair dark. And I've always had trouble with my voice.

With dark hair, I have a better base to stand on, in order to speak confidently and loudly.

People take me more seriously when I have darker hair than when it's blonde. I don't know if that's just my projection of my image of myself, or if they actually take me more seriously, listen to me, and do what I say?

If you can harness that ability to change how you look, to empower how you feel? That's the biggest power.

joanne

Once I was diagnosed with cancer and found out what treatments I would need, the first thing that went through my mind was: I can't lose my hair.

I absolutely cannot lose my hair.

I could deal with the surgeries and the chemotherapy. But the thought of being bald and not having any hair was the most frightening and terrifying.

I didn't want people to look at me differently. I didn't want to have to explain or have people pity me.

I think that without hair, I would have lost a big sense of identity, physically and emotionally.

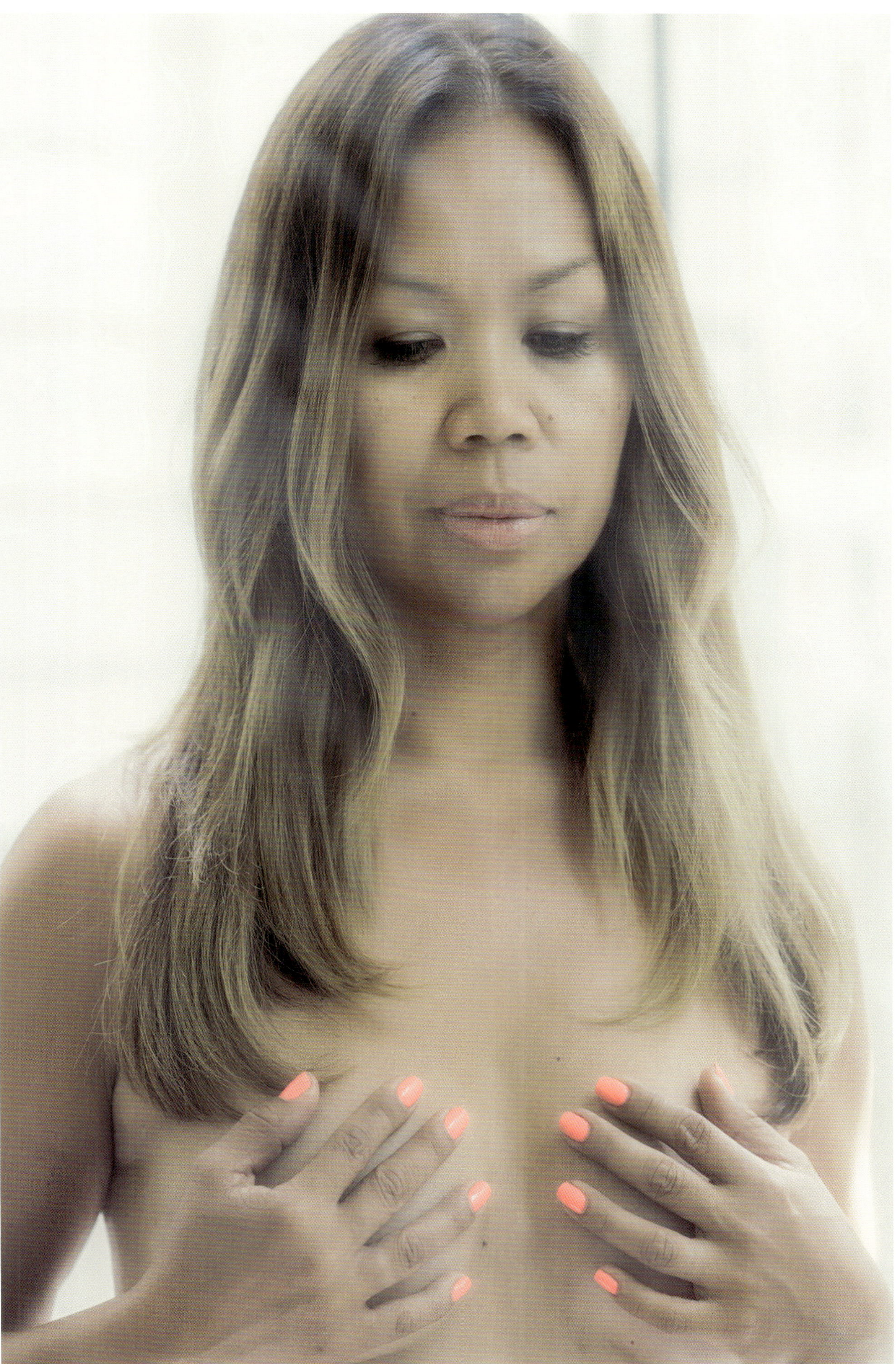

naomi

I used to be what they called a dirty blonde, but now it's white. I know there are women my age who wear wigs. I never considered it. I don't go out enough. I just brush it and go. I think if people don't like to look at me, then they don't have to. The empty space bothers me. That's all. You can see my skin. I cover it up the best I can.

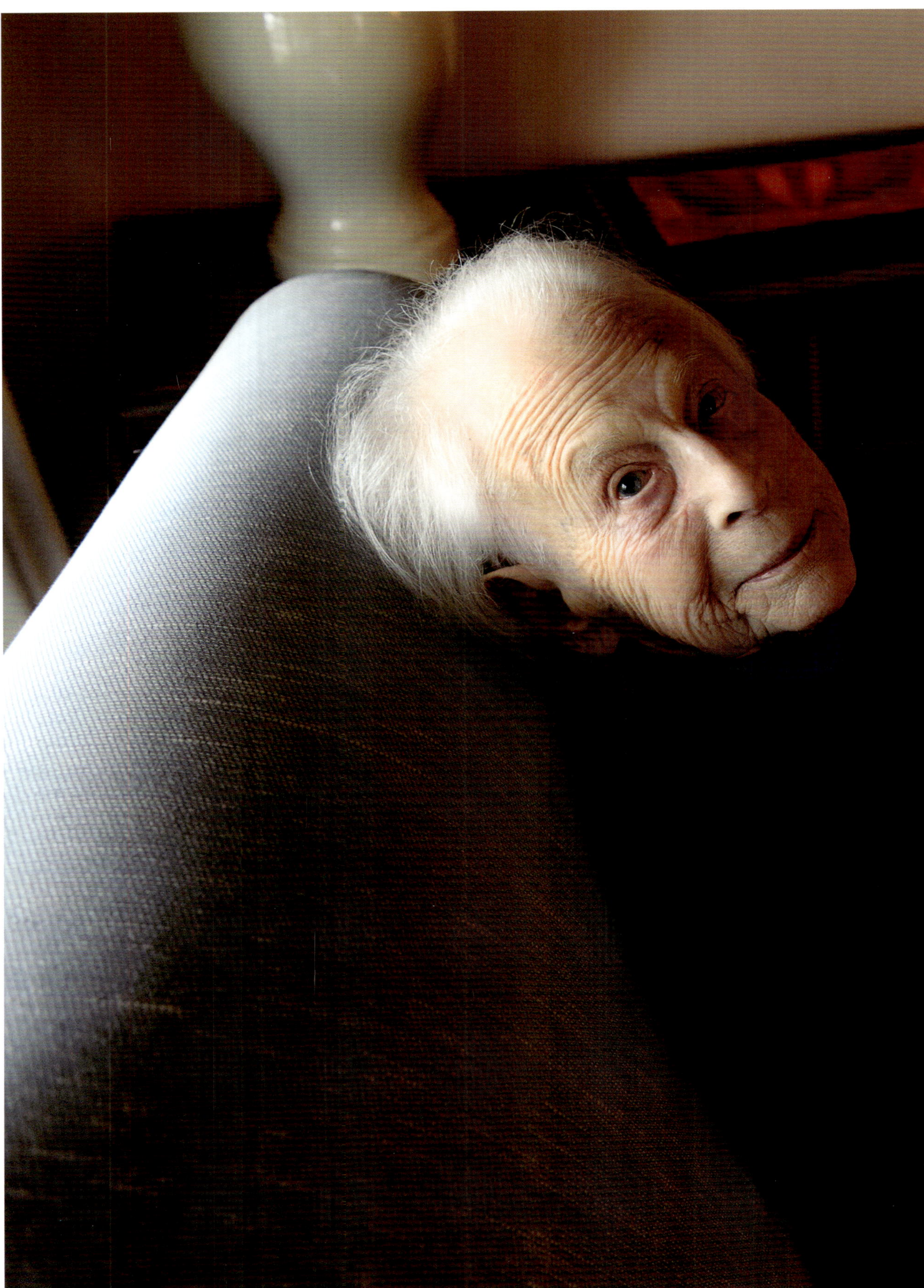

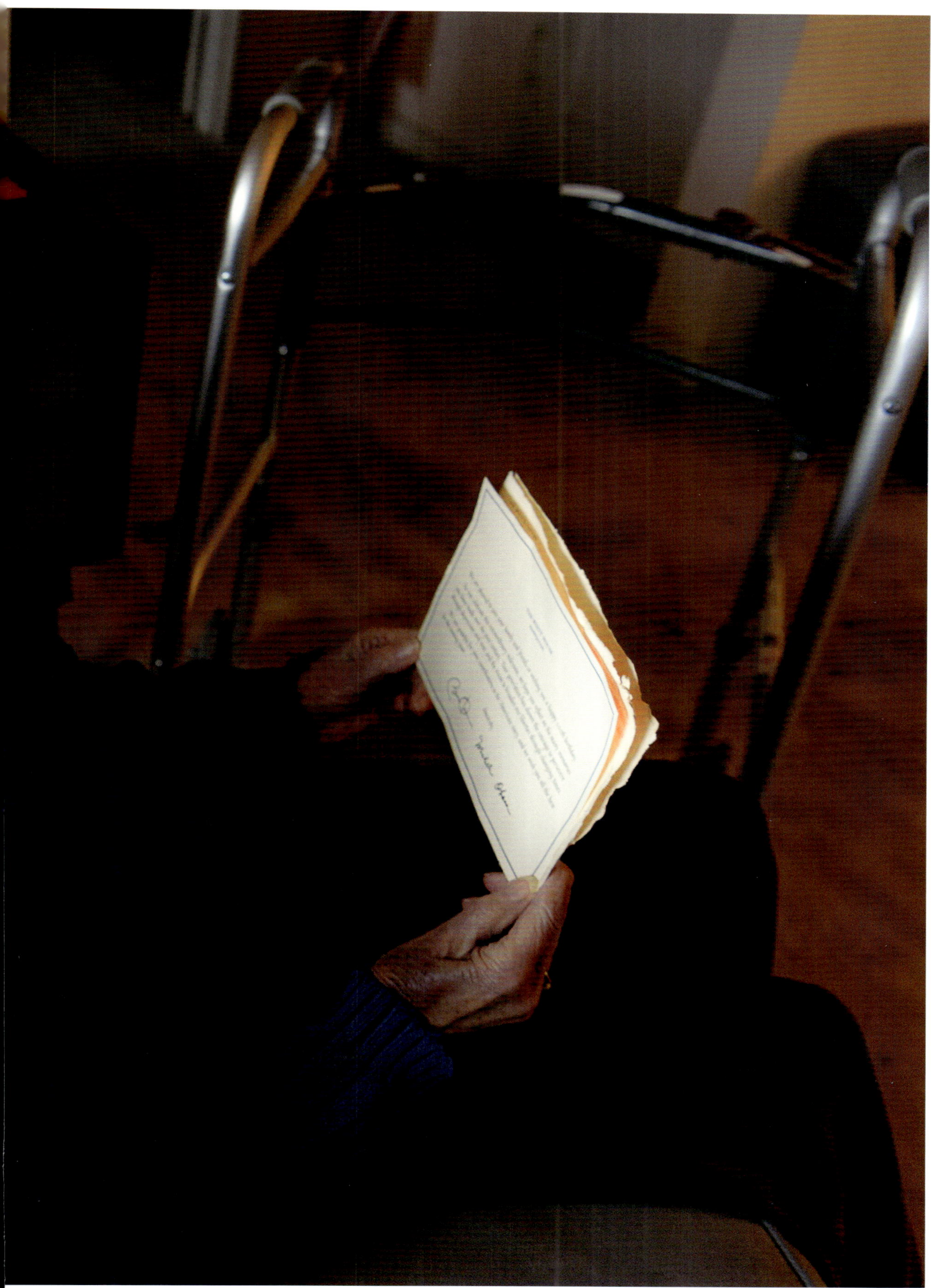

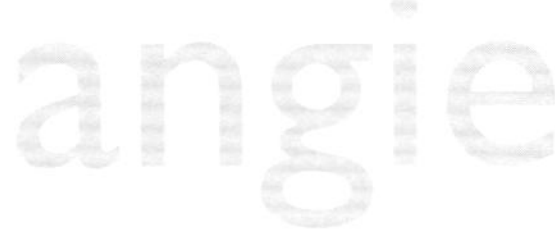

People used to come up to me and want to touch my hair. My mom kept it really long with severe bangs, like a cape. I used to resent the comments because they covered up people's interest in who I really was.

My ego was centered around my intelligence, so when people would comment on my hair, it felt like they weren't taking me seriously. I lived like that for a long time, out of fear of my parents because I was obedient, and didn't know I was allowed to be an individual. Eventually, I cut off at least a foot and a half of hair, and then burst out with who I really was.

I knew it would form a new identity and help me start again. It also removed the weight of my childhood and felt really good. It was like going to the ocean and letting it rip.

I found a whole new perspective on life, and it felt like I was levitating because all that hair was such a weight. I realized it was very consuming, all the time it took to shampoo and dry it, and I was thrilled to be done with all of that.

As I've grown, I realized you get your identity through other ways, and I feel confident about who I am as an artist and musician. My style has become part of the playfulness and the art, instead of a reflection of my ego.

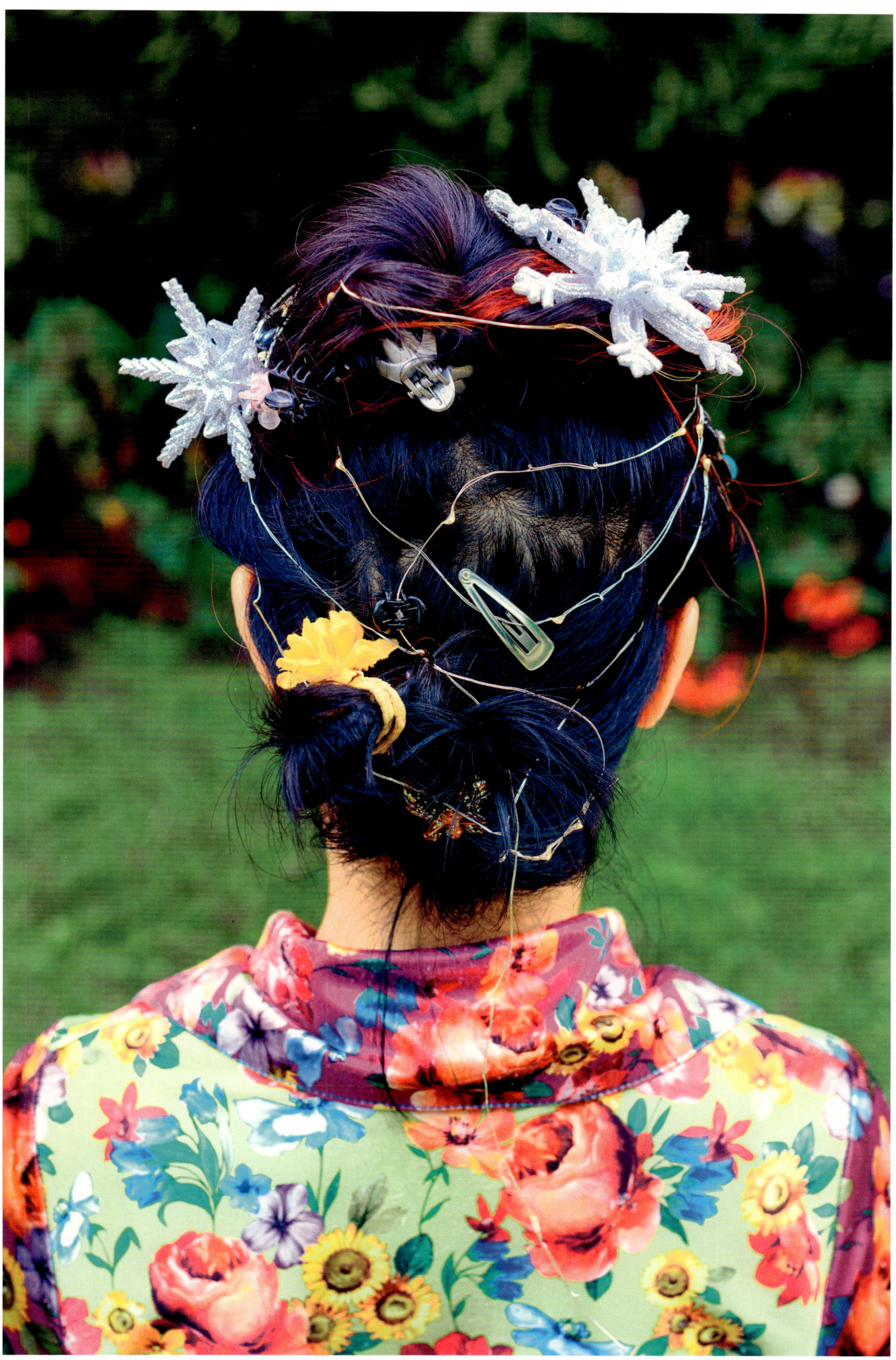

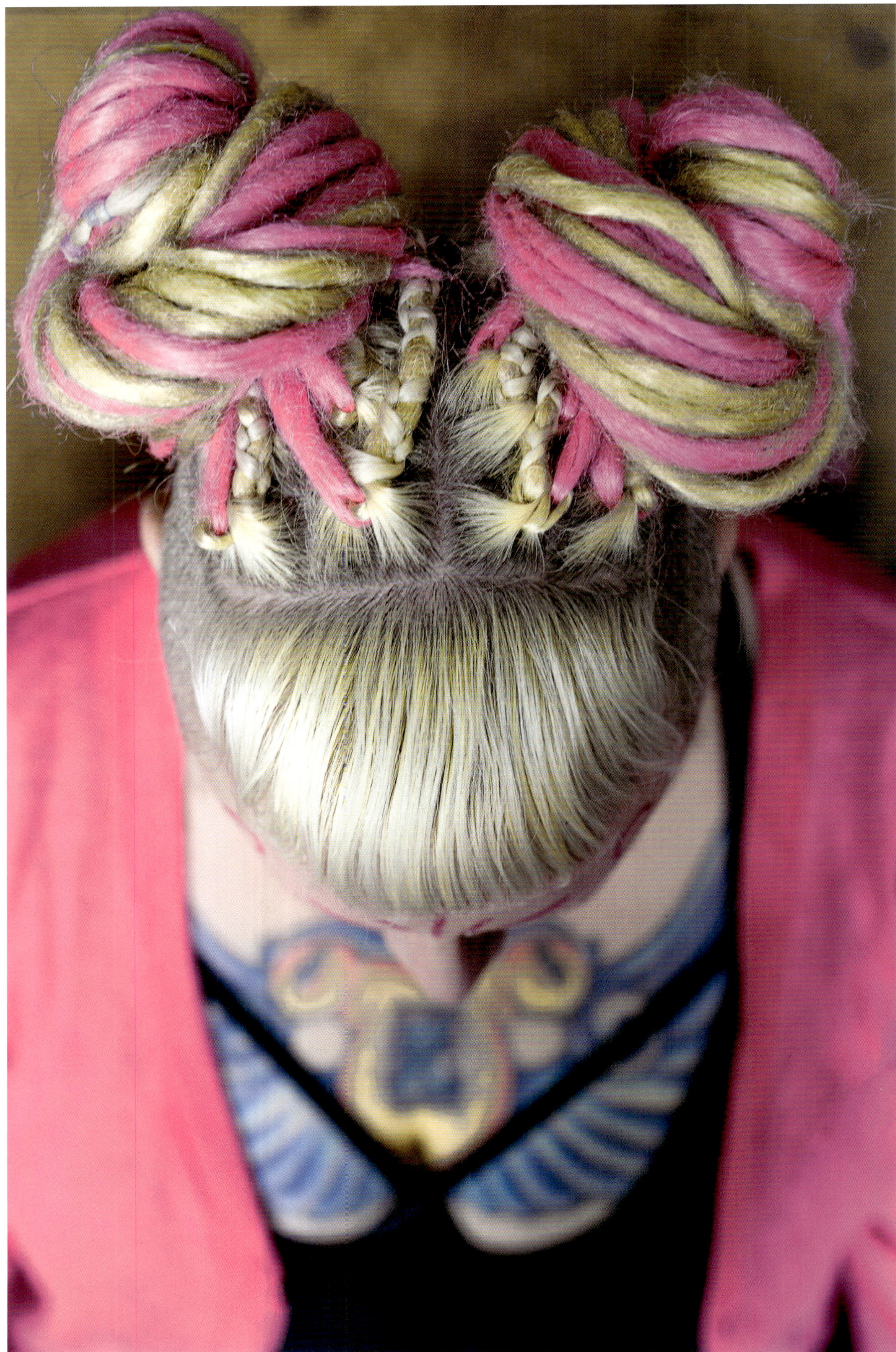

misha

Hair is actually a HUGE identifier for me.

I am an old punk rocker and hair was how we expressed ourselves. We shaved our heads, or did it up in funny colors. Our hair identified our difference.

I felt different on the inside for so very long and didn't fit in, no matter how much I tried. I have actually cut my hair to try to fit in, and have attempted to make myself look more like the people around me, hoping it would connect me in some way.

When I cut the hair off, it actually was very freeing. I felt like, "No, this IS me. I'm strange; my hair is strange. If you're going to hate me, hate me. At least you won't hate me for who I'm pretending to be to please you."

The pink has been the most successful. People treat me differently when I have pink hair. It's very welcoming, as if the color itself draws people.

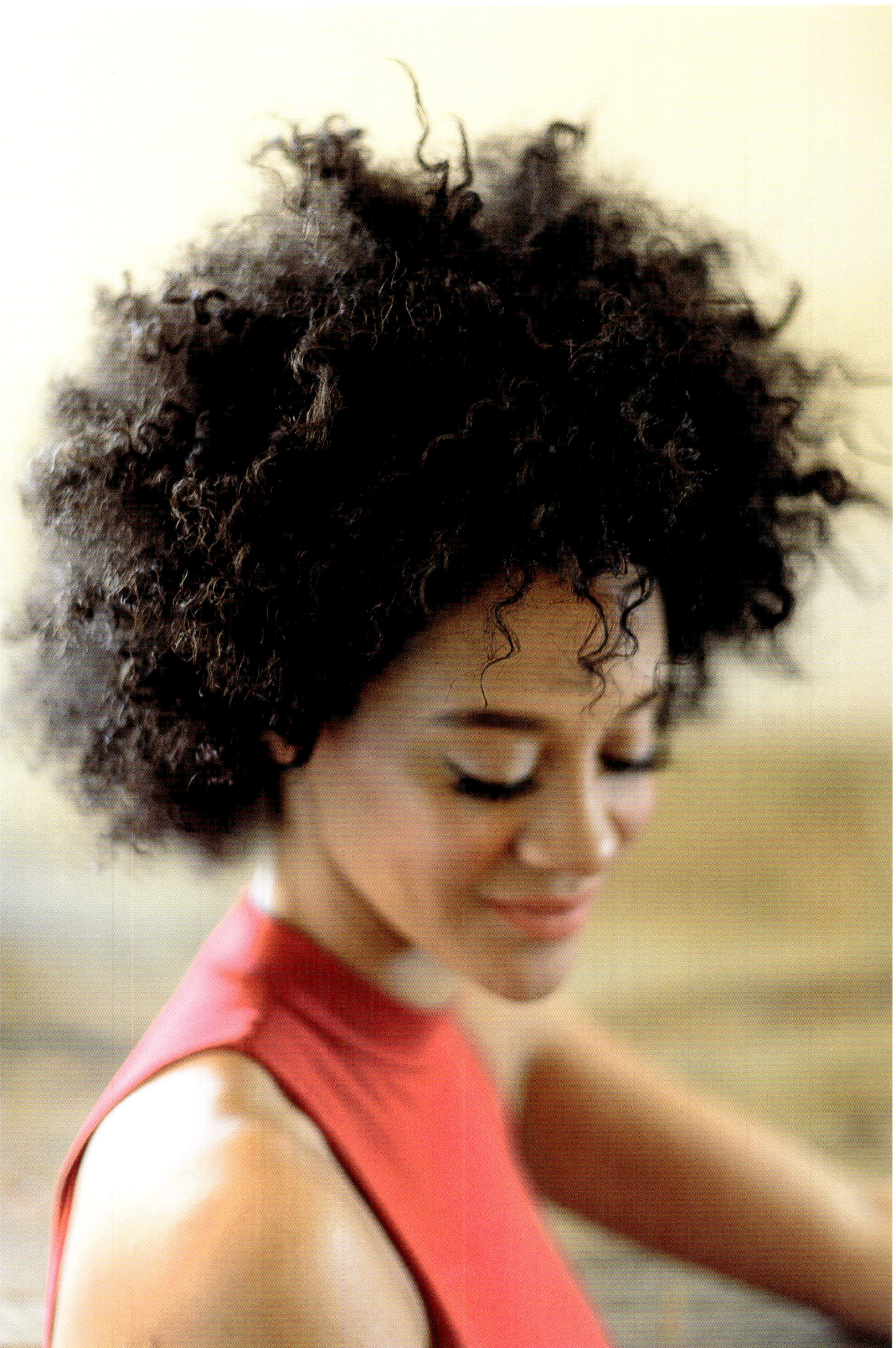

tiffany

This is actually my first time wearing my hair natural. Since the age of 15 I had been wearing a weave. There's an ease to it. You can just wake up and go.

It's not about perfection. It makes me look like I am fine the way I look, and fine the way I am. I feel really stripped down, which is nice, because I'm not trying to look like anyone else. I just feel free, like I've changed, which helped me be ready to go natural. With the weave, it was like putting on a costume. With this I feel authentic.

samantha

I've had a problem with my hair my whole life.

I had long hair, and it defined me in a way that other things didn't, because I was a chubby child. My hair was my "crowning glory," but when I was 5 or 6, my hair was chopped off into a Buster Brown haircut. It was blunt and very unattractive, and I never got over it. Even at that age I felt the loss.

The short haircut didn't do anything to enhance my feelings about myself. To exacerbate the situation, there was an old man down the street that molested both my sister and me.

I had to testify, and it was a very traumatic experience. So I grew up feeling ugly and unattractive, and my hair was always an issue. My ears stuck out, no matter what I did with my hair.

It's now shorter than it's been almost my whole life. I think I look better than with the straggly hair, and somehow my ears peeking through don't bother me so much.

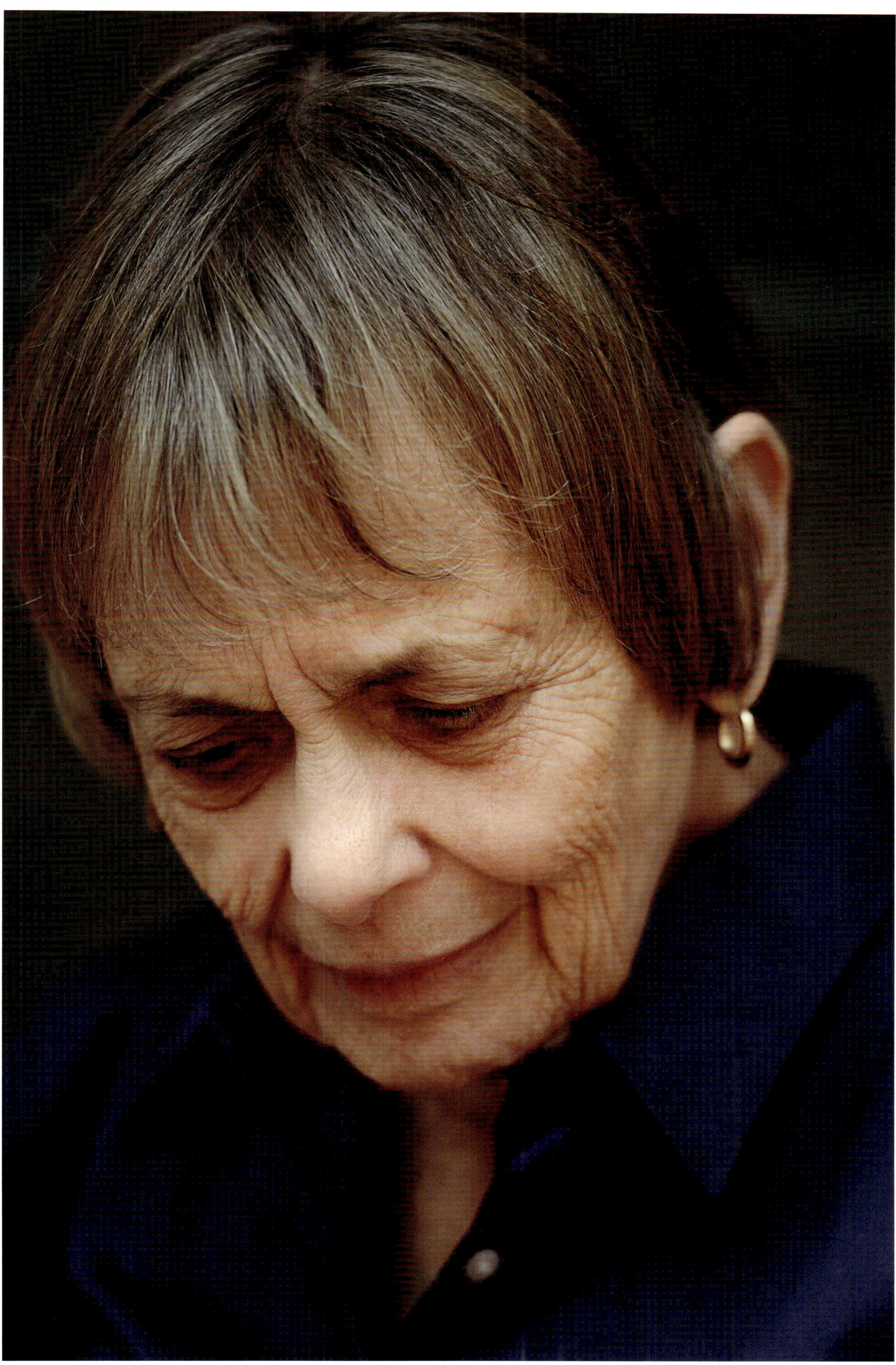

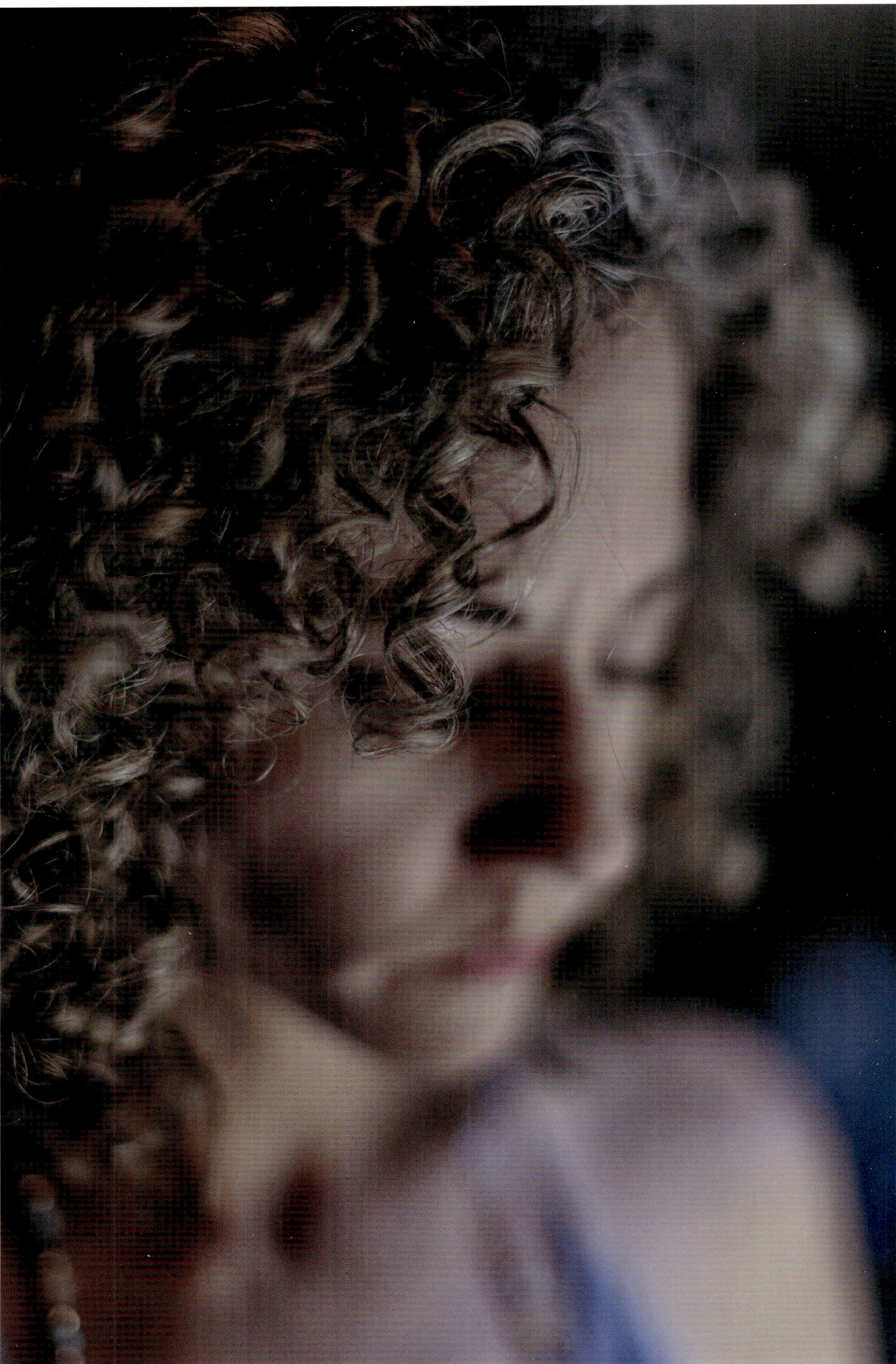

I wasn't born with my hair this curly; it happened because of medication. When I was 15, I had a grand mal seizure, and the medication they put me on was one dose too high.

Half of my hair fell out.

I don't remember the day it started to grow back curly. I just know that all of a sudden, it was there. I guess that's the only way I can put it: that I had very curly hair at the top of my head.

I had a Brillo pad.

I was scared. It was already enough to be me. I was so used to being different. Once it was under control, I was fine.

carolyn

Seeing my daughters go gray, dealing with their hair the way I had, I finally accepted who I was. I realized, seeing my daughters so beautiful – all of them- that I was actually beautiful too, but I had to feel it myself. I had an epiphany. I took off the mask, freed myself and embraced everything: my aging, my creativity, my mistakes, my life, and my hair. It's now slightly brunette but mostly gray with an inch of blonde just waiting to be cut off.

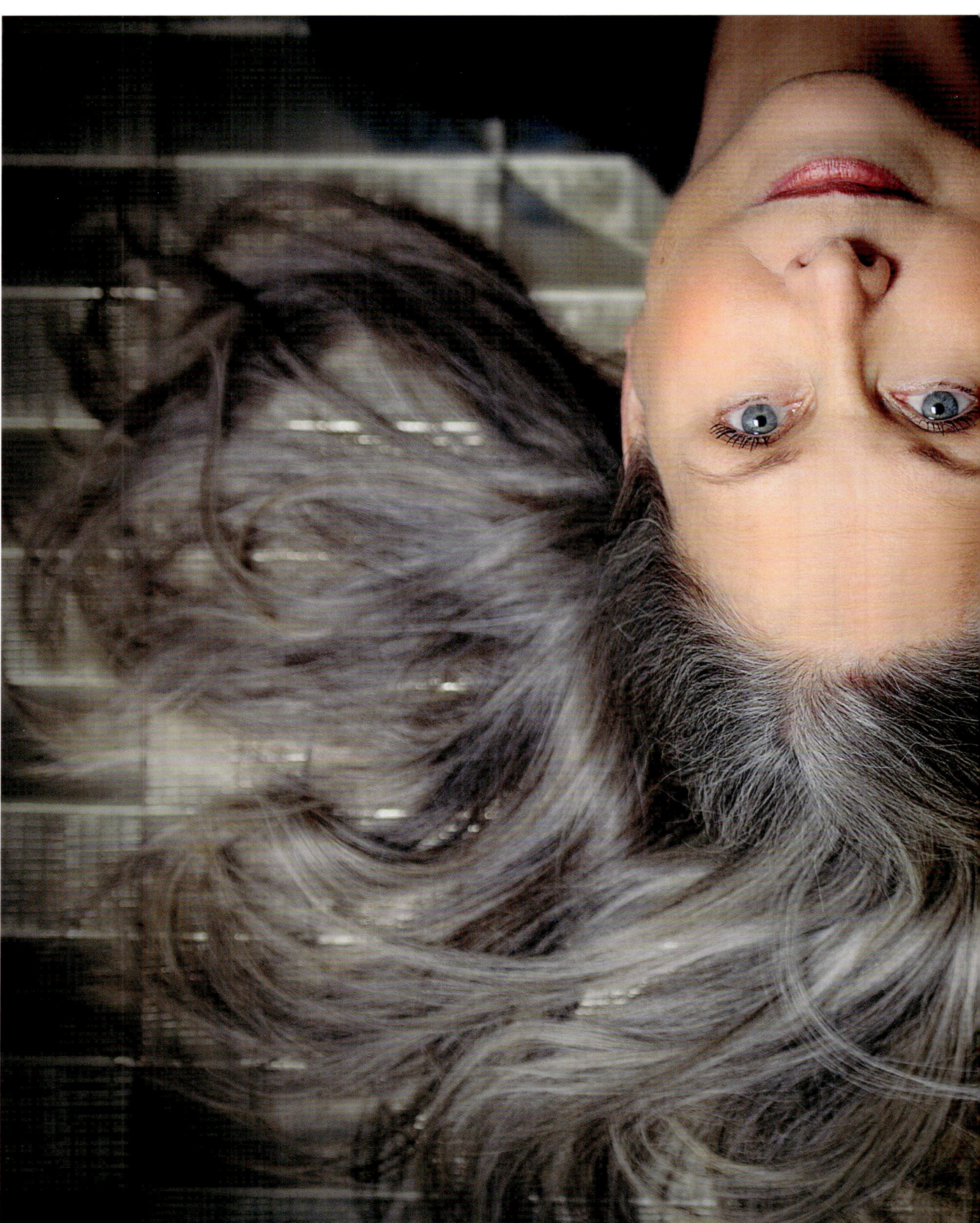

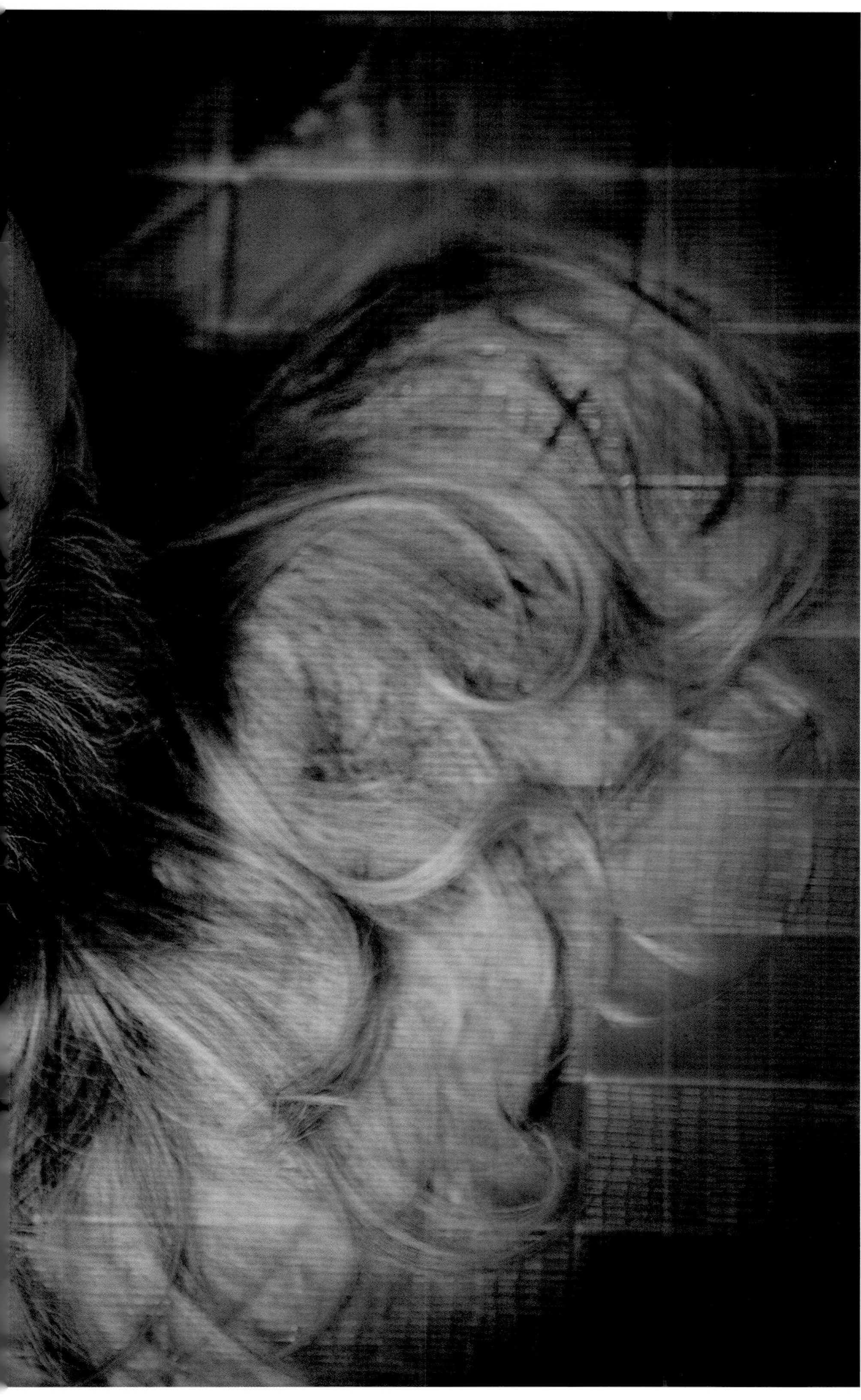

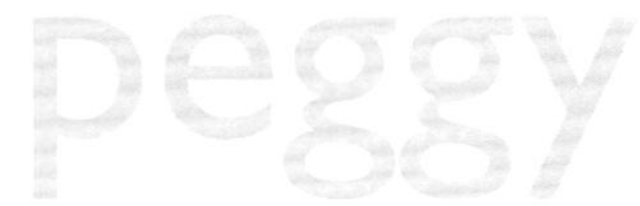

I used to work in the hair care industry so I had to look good. If I showed my roots, it had to be colored right away. Every four weeks I was in the chair for two hours at a time.

It was a long process.

I went through the grey process, which took about a year and a half. I was wearing a hat every day, then I just kept cutting it until there was no more color left.

And then this is what I came up with. This is my hair color.
I cannot believe how much energy I put into my hair color. Once I stopped coloring it, I was like, "I'm free. I'm free."

When I'm with somebody now, I can be with them. I'm not worried about what I look like. I know they're just seeing me.

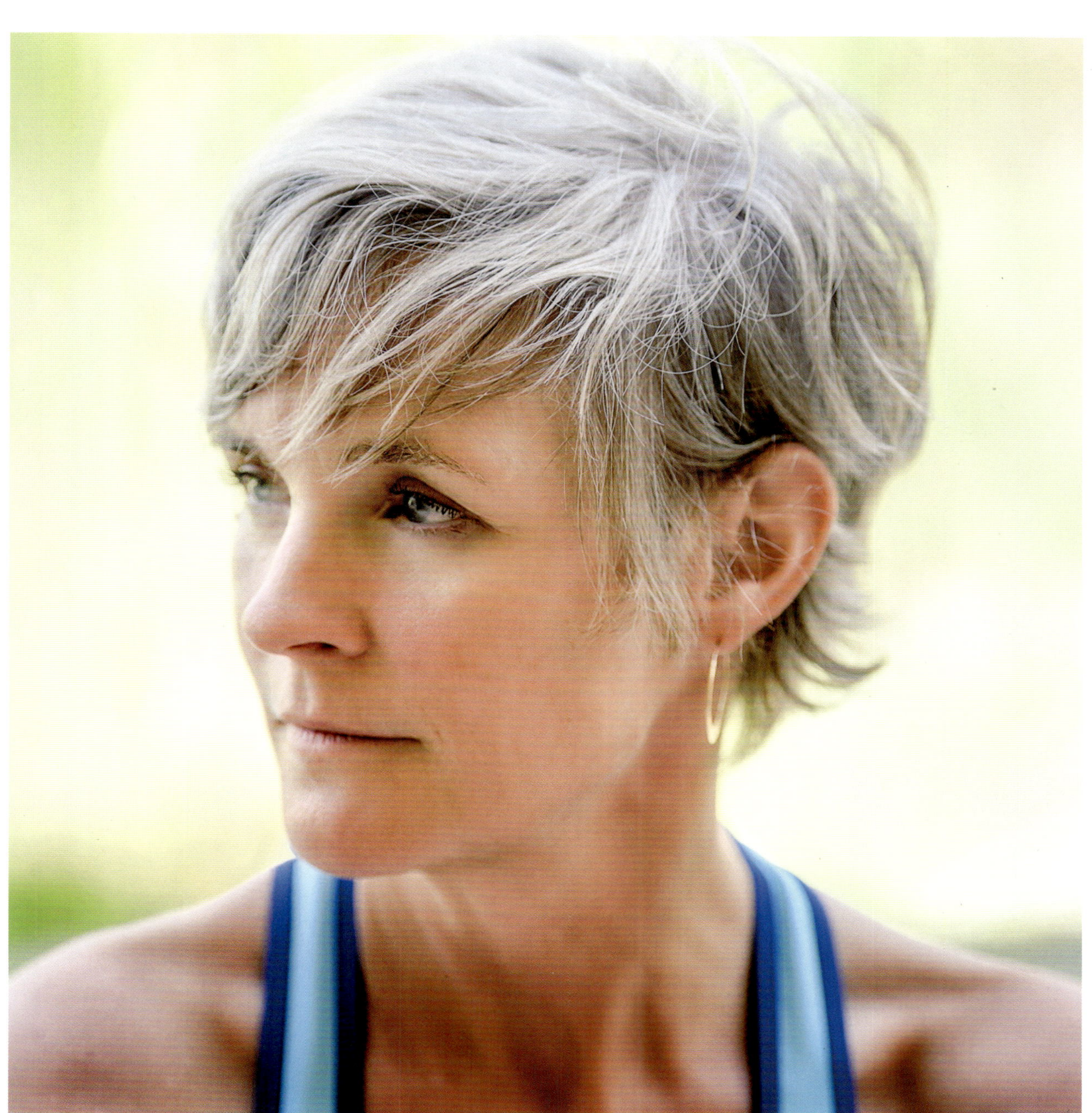

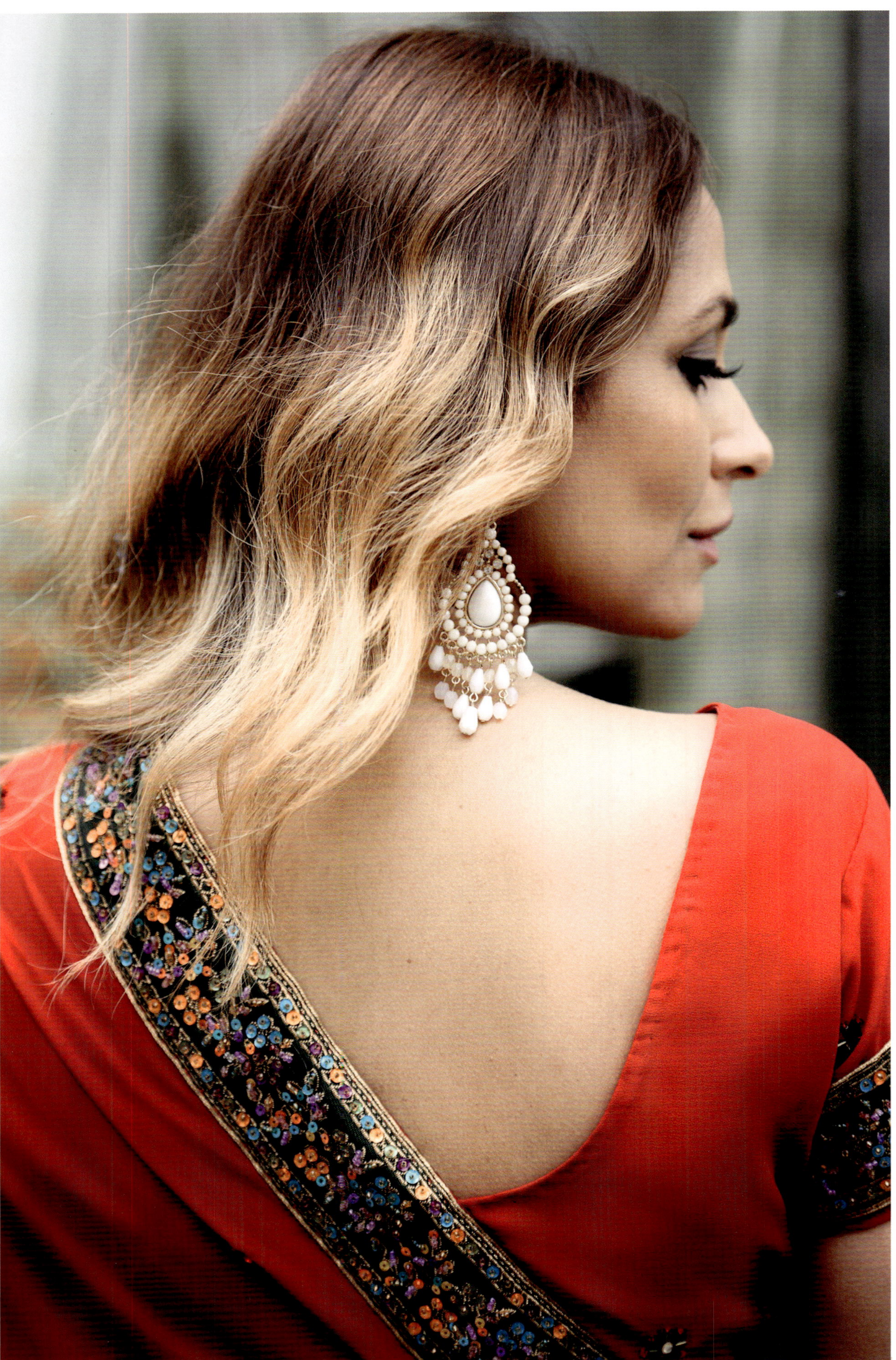

archna

I like having ethnic ambiguity. I reveal what I want to reveal about myself. I could be from anywhere because I'm a brown girl. No matter how light my hair is, I'll still be a brown girl.

My hair is mixed hair. My mom is Japanese and my dad is Black. And I have curly, wavy, crazy hair. Growing up, just like my hair, it's a mixed emotion. I appreciate it now, but when I was a kid, I definitely wanted something I didn't have.

All the traits inside of me are represented by my hair. This is my DNA.

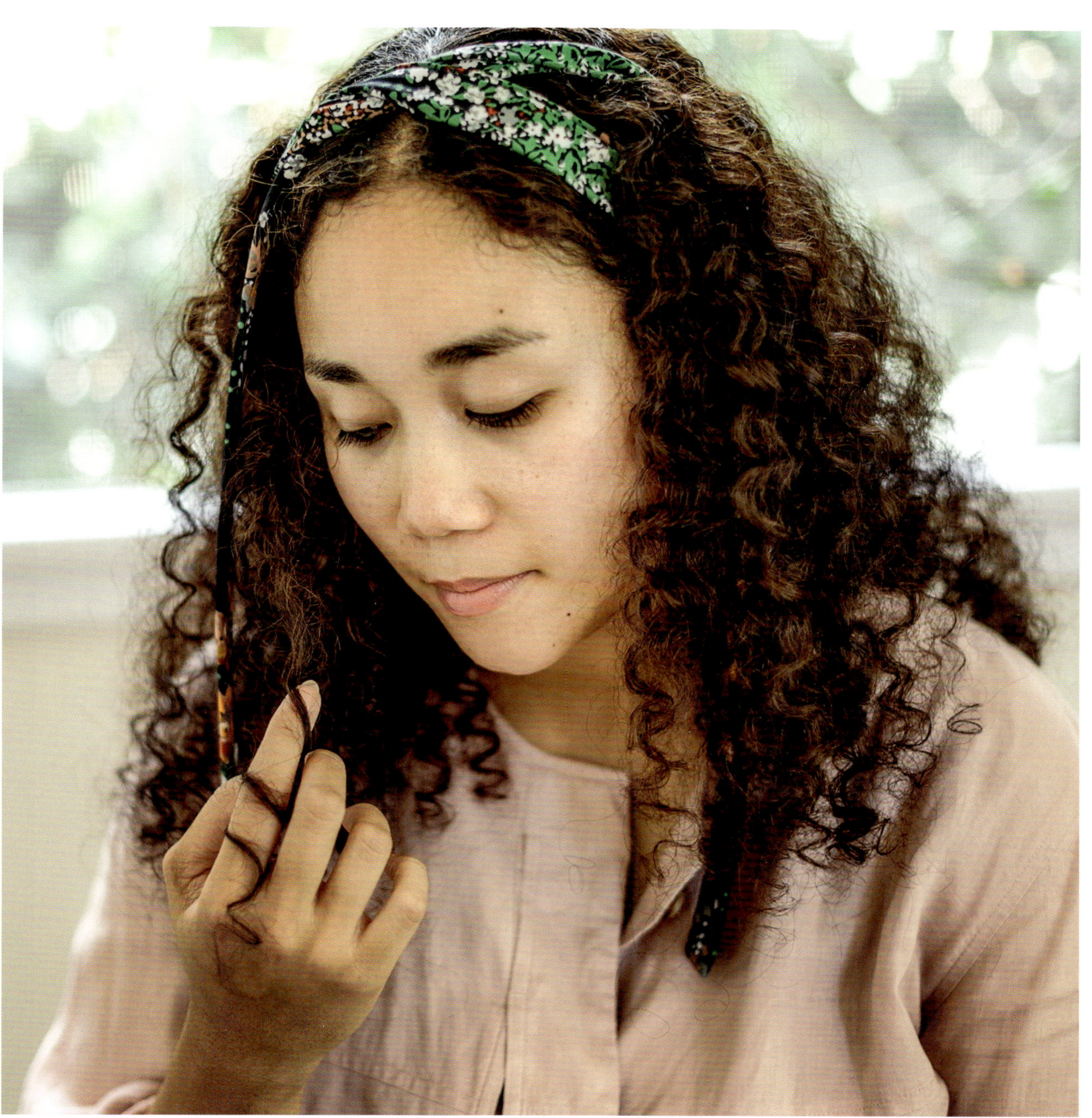

lauren

I'm always changing.

Some days I want short hair, and some days I want long hair. One day I want red hair, one day I want black.

I wear wigs all the time because I love changing my hair.
It's not like I'm ashamed of my hair. I just love having different hairstyles, because I feel like my personality is fun and different, and I want to try new things. Changing hairstyles is just a way for me to express myself.

I've always been like that.

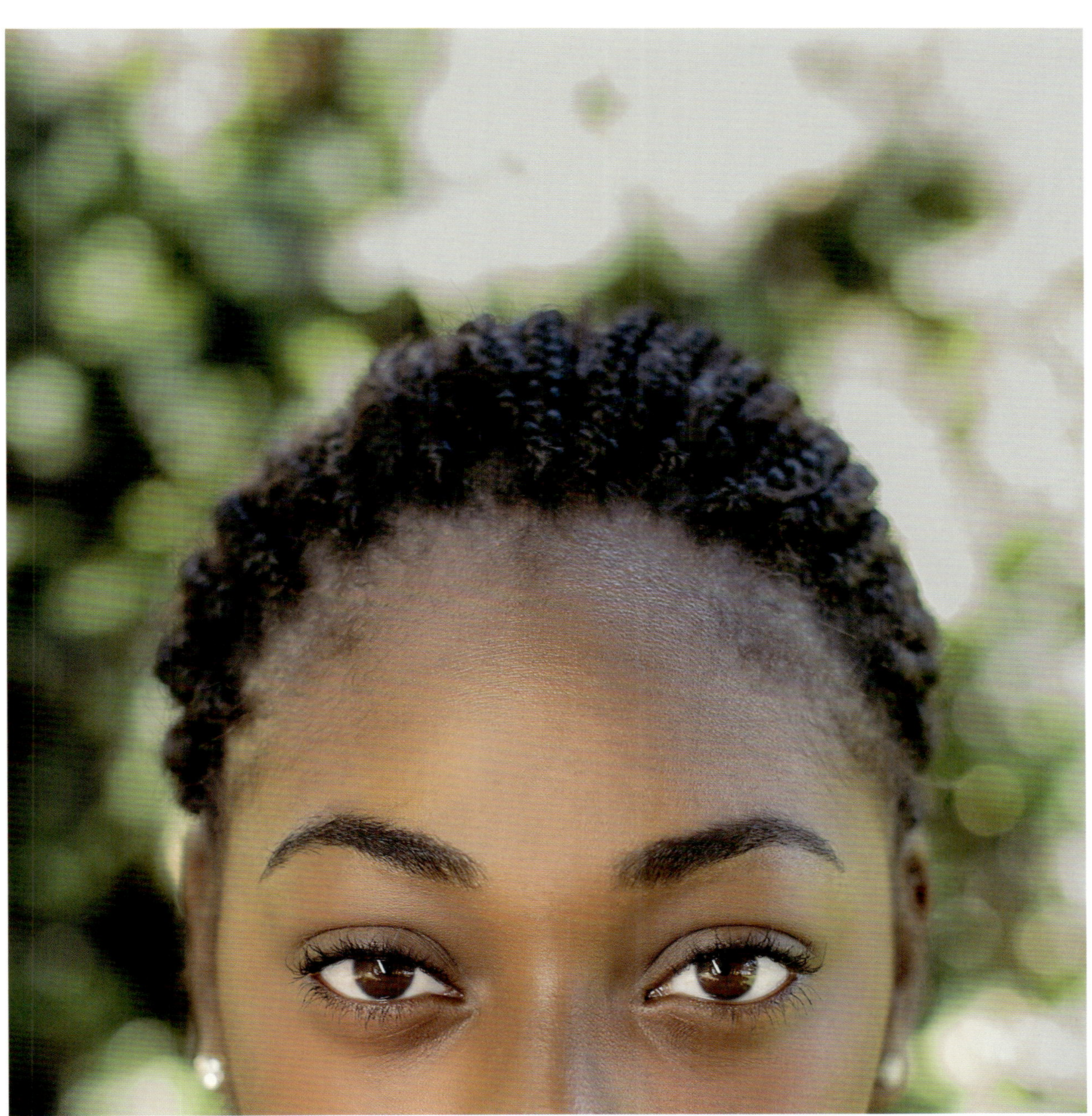

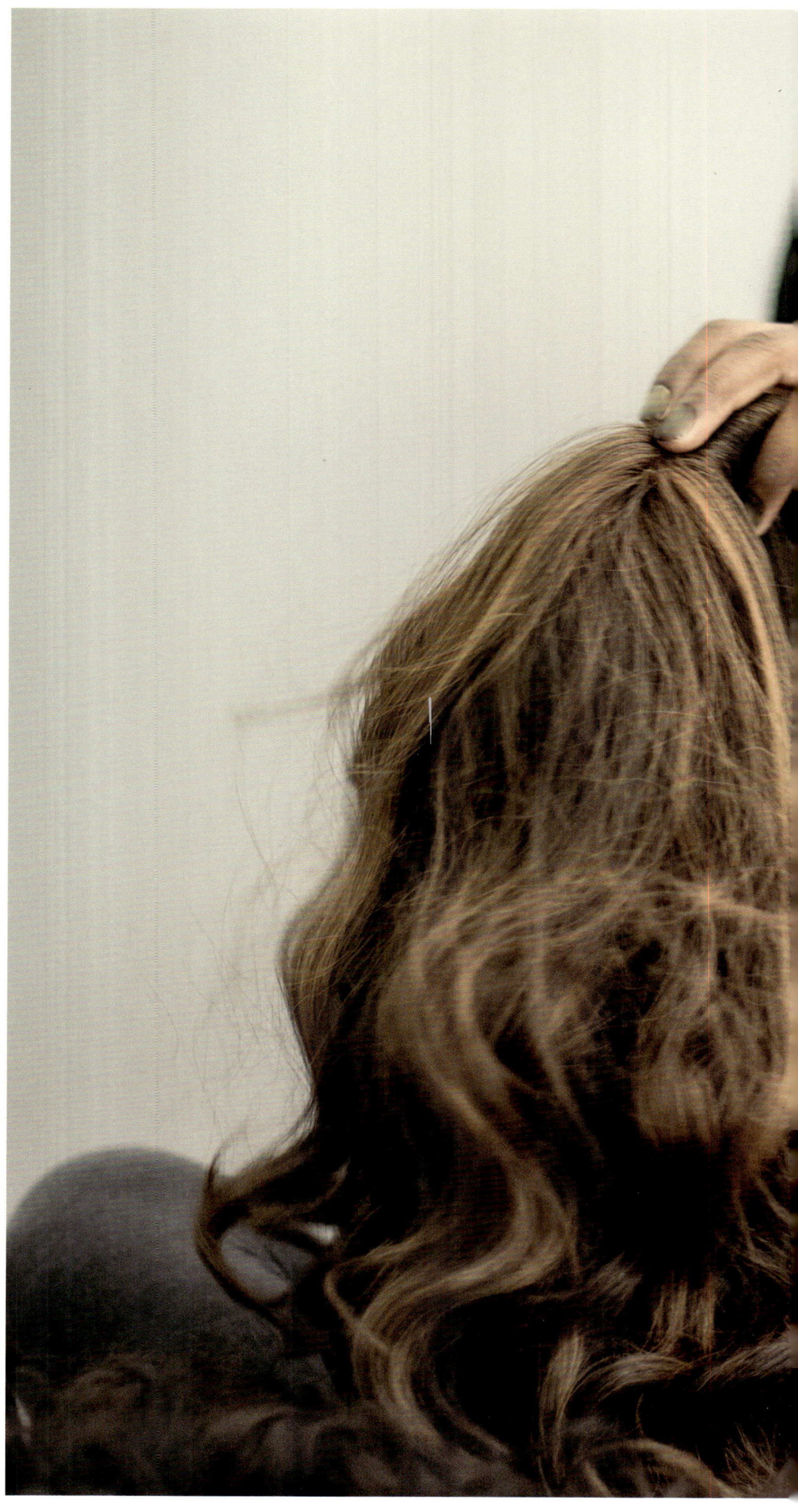

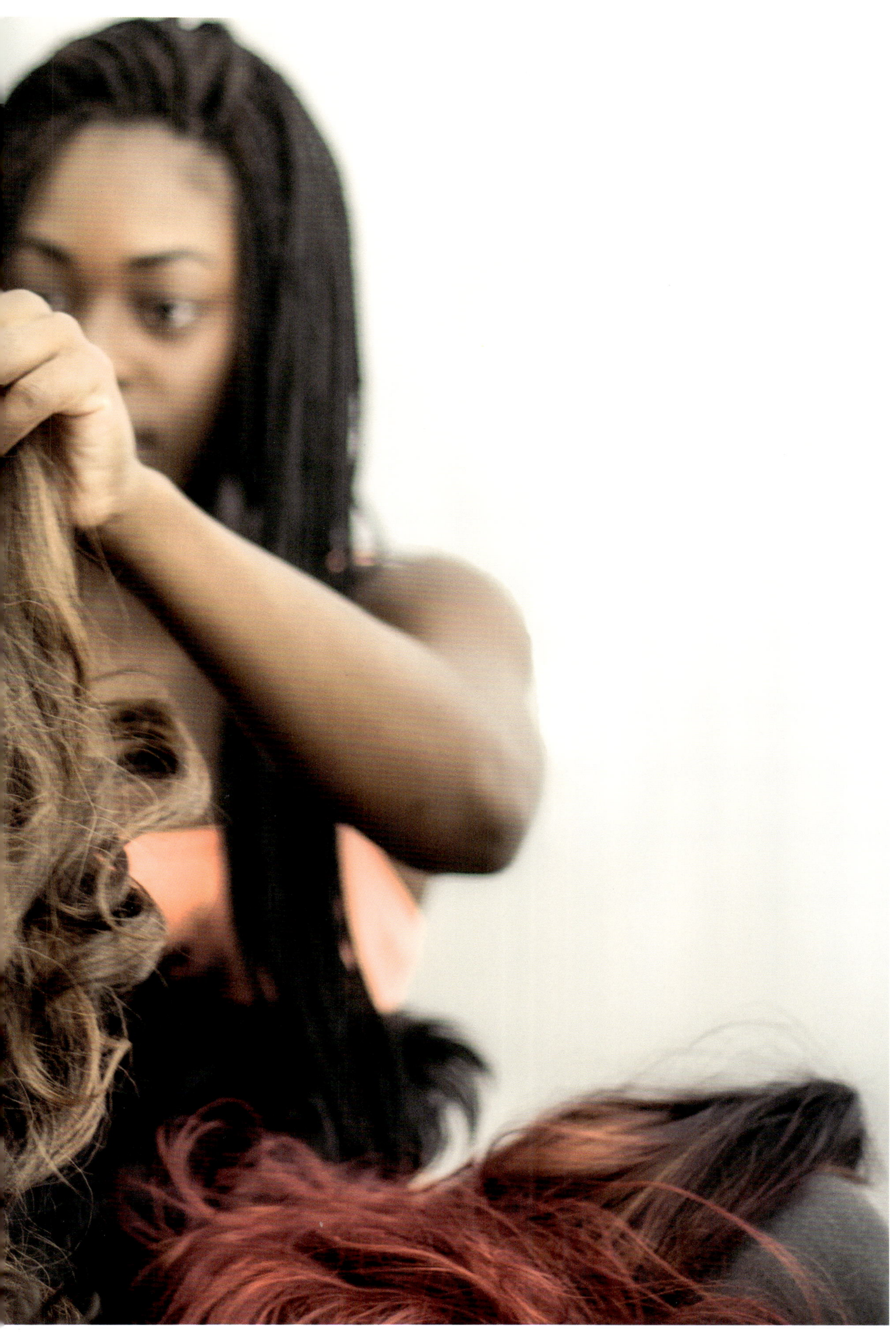

lila

I donated my hair to "Locks of Love." To me, it's just dead skin cells growing out of your head. If you mess it up, you can always fix it.

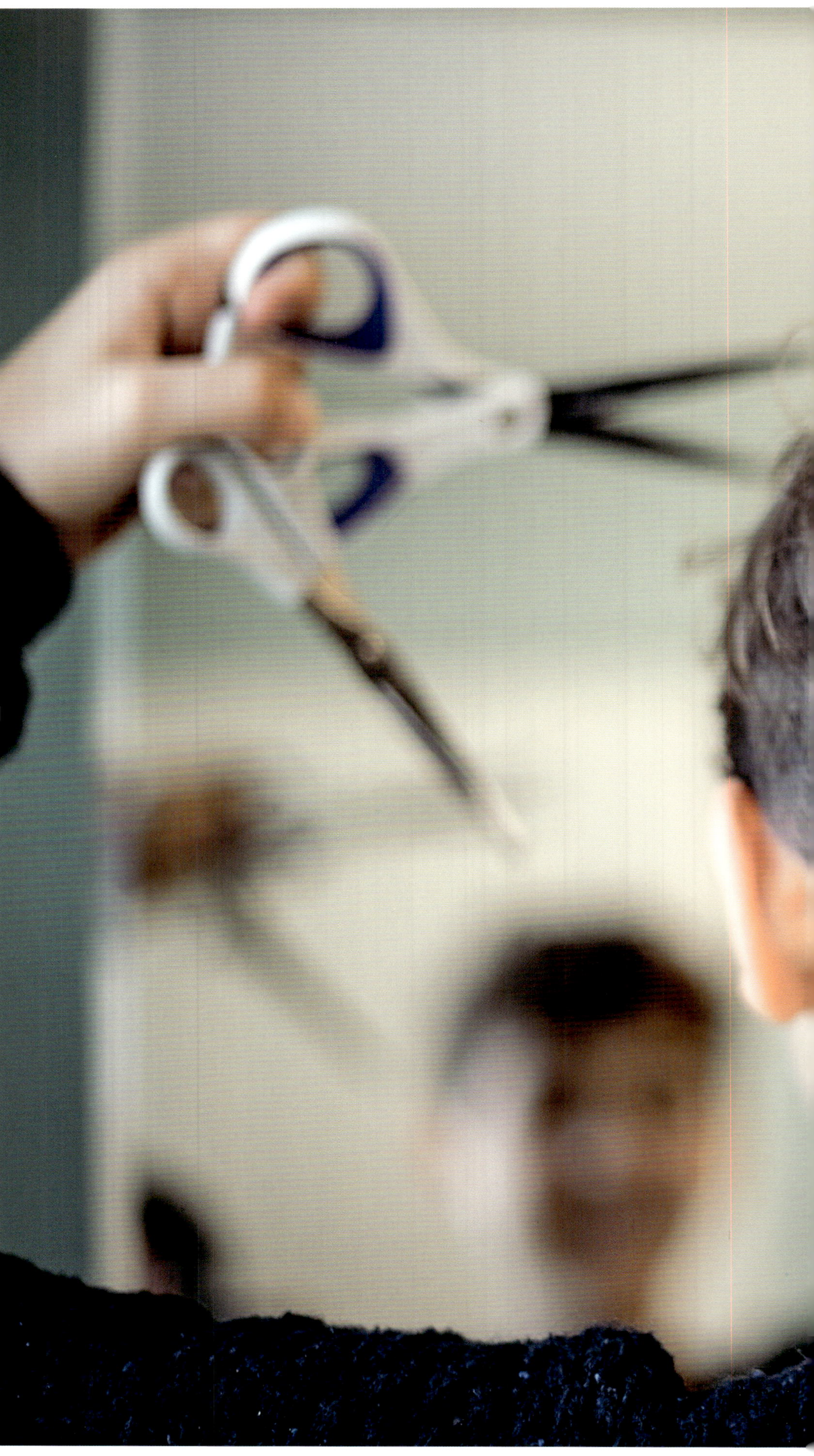

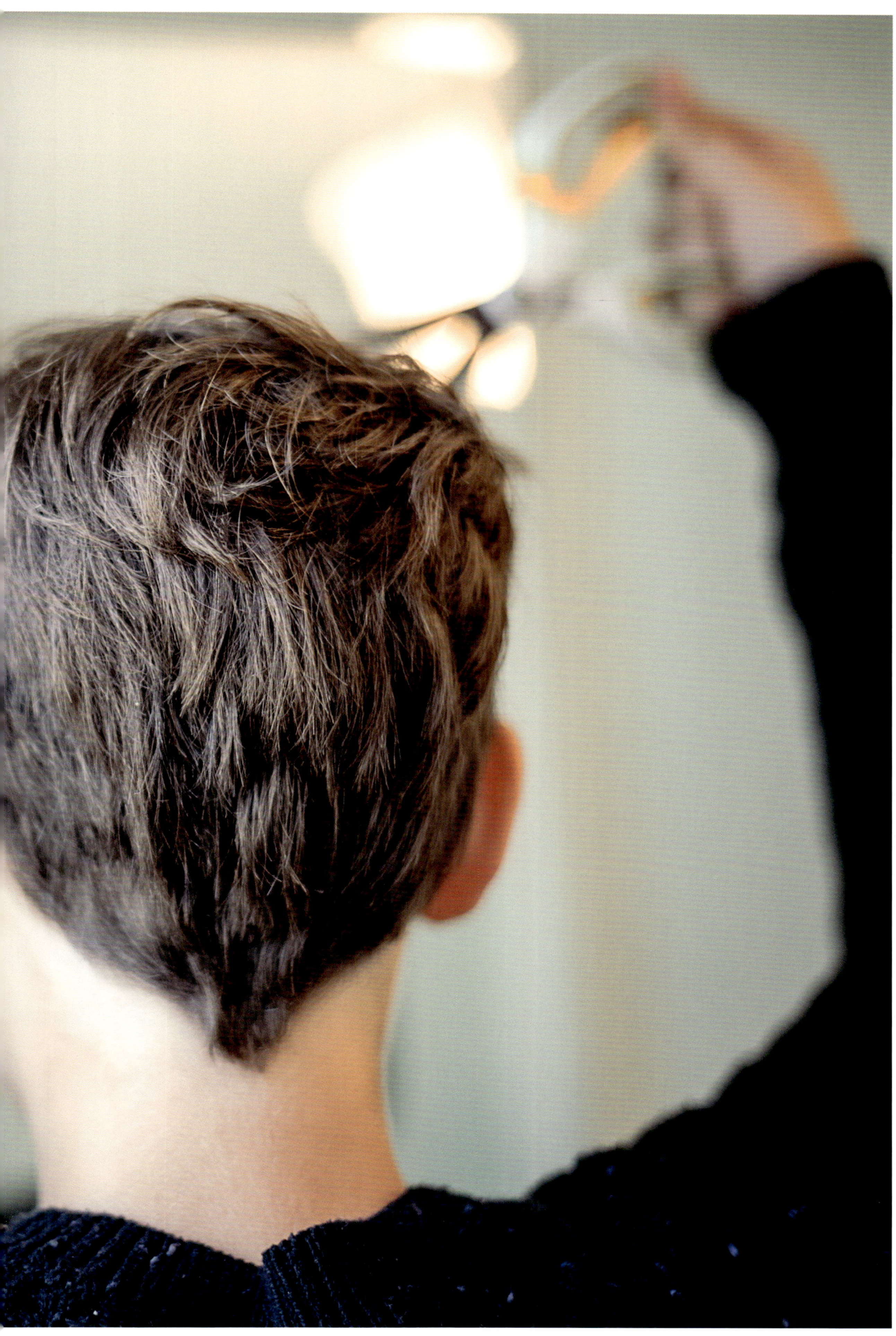

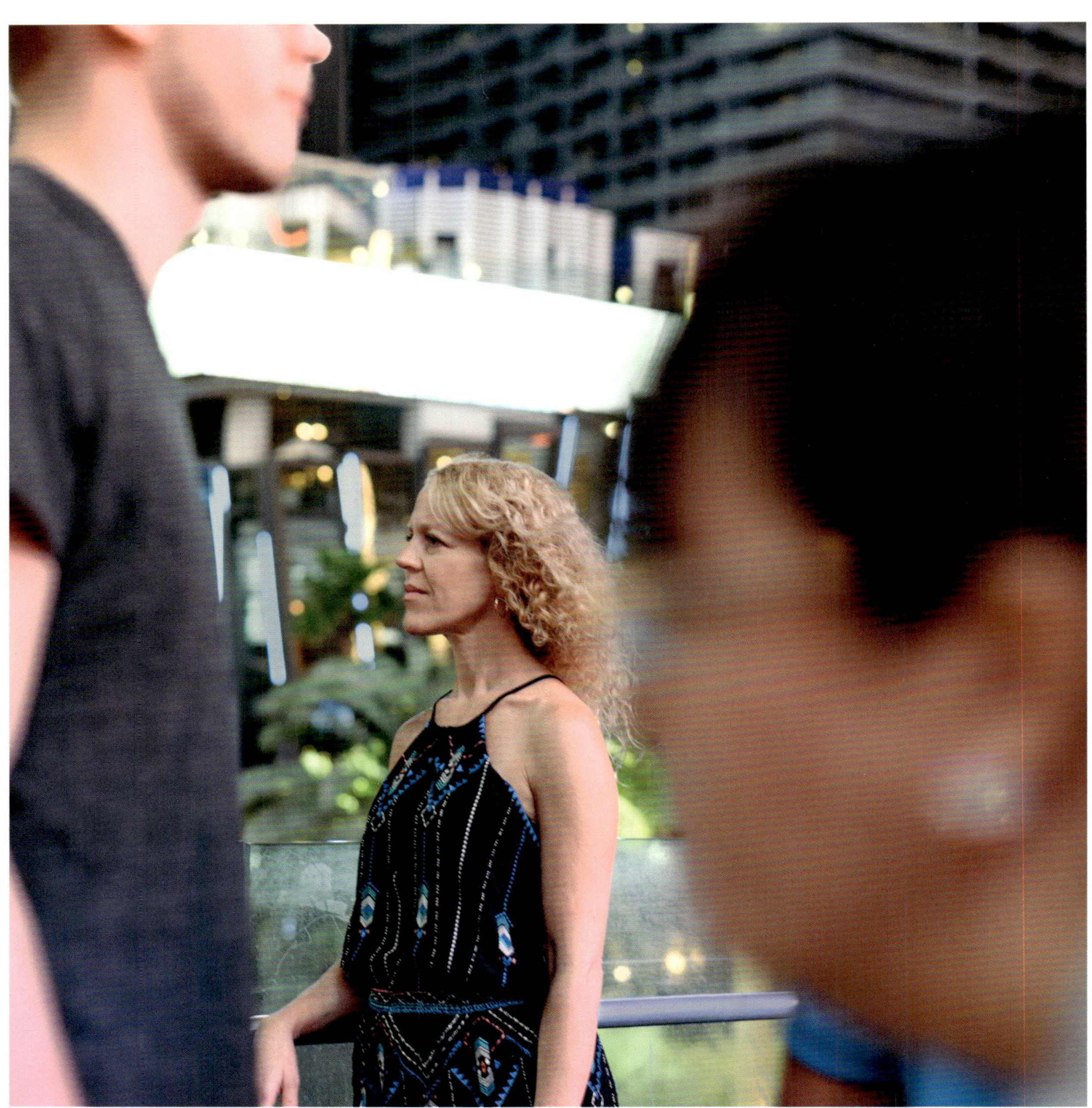

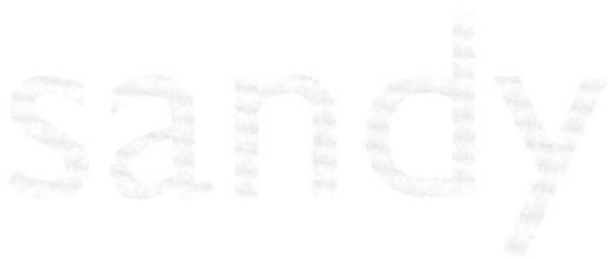

I was born completely bald and my hair didn't grow in until I was about three. Then, it grew in little short corkscrews, and it took a long time for my hair to grow down, so it was always up in a little blonde afro.

My mom always thought that to control curly hair you need to keep it short, so when it started to grow longer, she would get it cut.
She always wanted me to look like Shirley Temple. I just had this little, curly mop.

I always hated my hair, and when I was young, people always mistook me for a boy. I wanted the princess hair, the Rapunzel hair.

When I'd go out with my mom, they'd be like, "Oh, what's your son's name?" When I was already, like, seven years old. I hated it, and felt invisible as a girl because I felt I looked like a boy.

Now I have a four-year-old daughter, and she also had no hair when she was born. Then it started growing in, and she has my hair.

I can't believe I ever hated it because it's so beautiful on her. I feel like those feelings I had about myself when I was young were not valid, now that I see it in my daughter. And I look forward to raising her where she can feel her identity. I don't want to impose what I want for her identity. I don't control that.

salma

The head scarf brings way more attention than you want.

In some ways, though, it's a good thing. Sometimes, you have the opportunity to change people's opinions. If you get the chance, and give them a chance.

I first started covering up in middle school. I did it for God, as a way to get closer to Him and to remember Him throughout my day. And then secondly, I did it for myself. The most critical part of this concept of hijab is the idea of modesty, so that your dealings with others are based on who you are and your personality rather than how you look. How do you carry yourself? How do you put yourself out there? How do you see yourself?

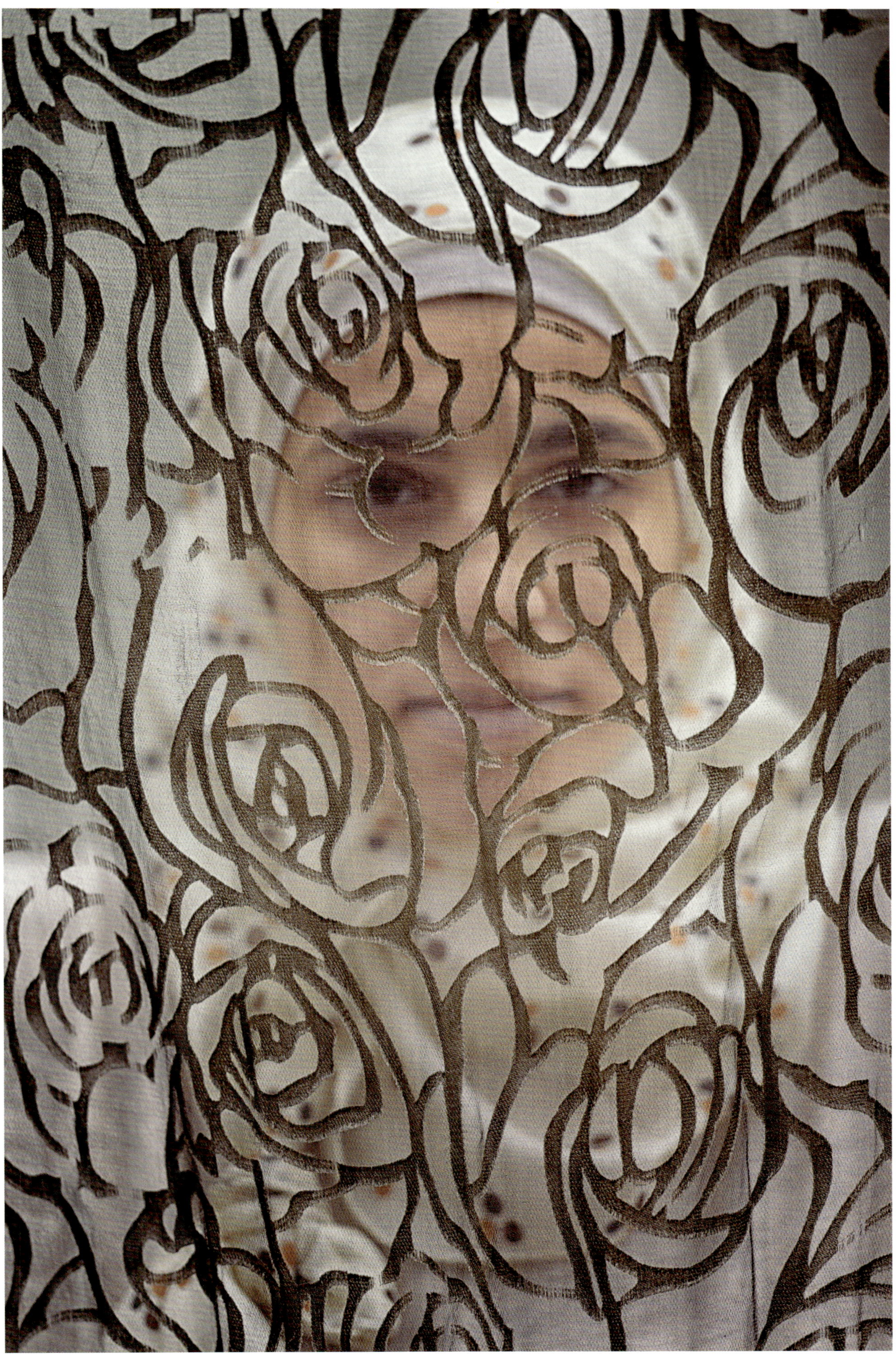

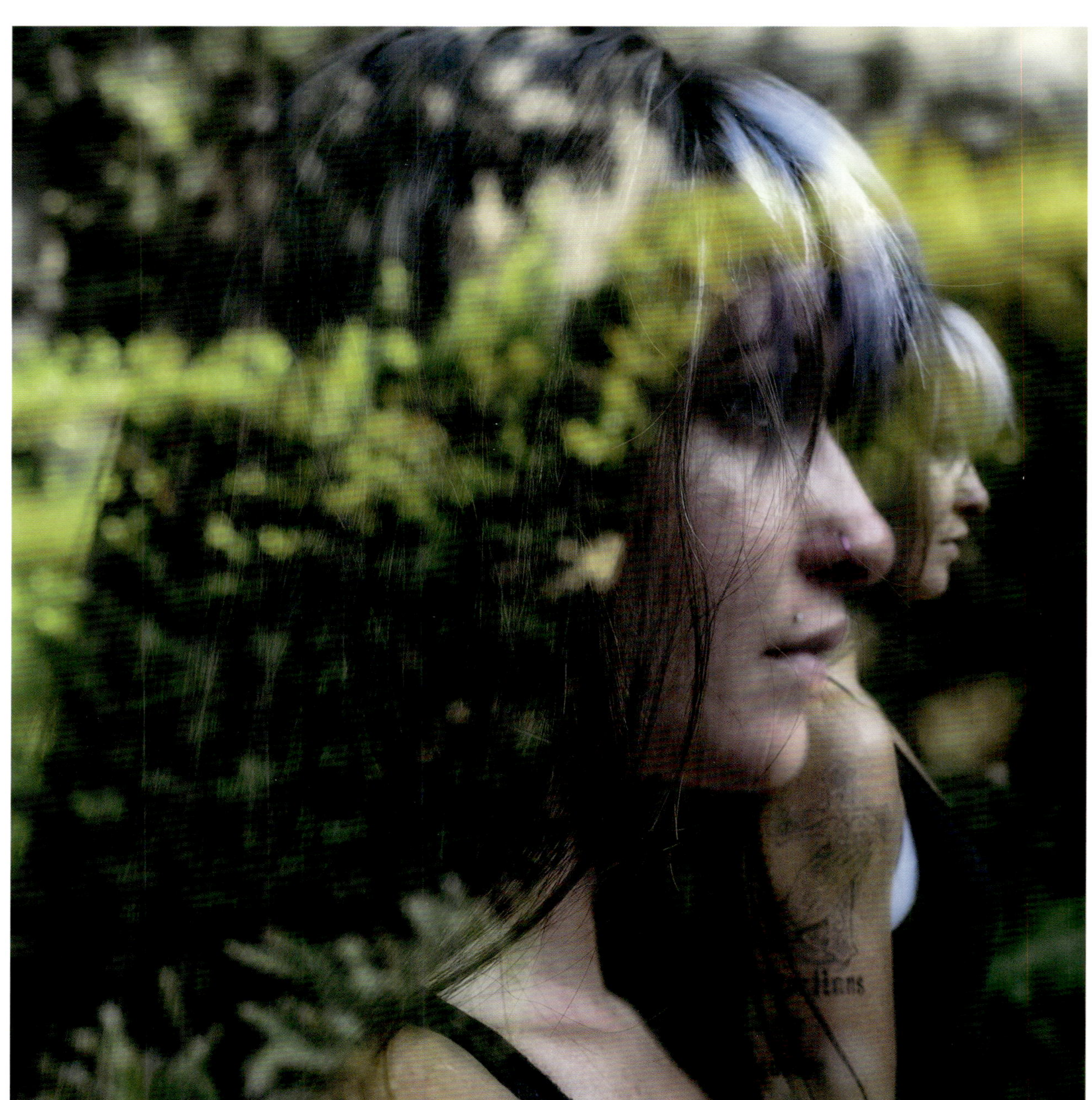

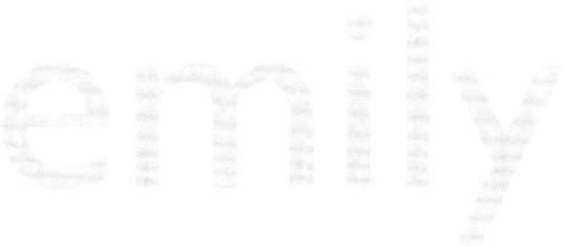

From way back when, women were taught to have long hair. All the magazines and social media have always taught us, "This is the way your hair should look." So when you go against something like that, everyone thinks it's wrong, even though it's just a personal preference. Nothing's wrong or right.

A lot of people in school just didn't get who I was. Through my experimental phases with my hair, it did bring on some negative attention. I definitely feel hair is very powerful and that's probably why I became a stylist. I wanted to help people feel good about themselves. It's always changing and growing. That's why I keep a job. So yeah, I love hair.

judith

I feel like I started standing out after I began coloring my hair. Before, I was medium height with medium brown hair and medium brown eyes. Medium can be a synonym for average. Afterwards, I started noticing in photographs that it was like lights from the heavens were shining upon my head, and I felt very special.

Since the change, my eyes have turned hazel, probably to accommodate my blonde hair.

I went to places where they'd make it a little brassy, and that didn't work. And the truth is there are intelligent-looking blondes, classy-looking blondes, and stupid-looking blondes, so finding the right blonde was difficult.

Sometimes you get it right; sometimes you don't. Coloring your hair is so common among women, I call it "the gilding." You have to sit with stuff on your hair for almost an hour, but it's always worth it, because you come out looking shimmery again. You're gilded.

Then everybody started getting highlights, and I see the girls these days. They start with highlights, and eventually they'll become like me. It's an epiphany, today, that perhaps coloring your hair sets you apart. Ironically, though, many of my friends have now become blonde. So when we go out, it's almost like I'm back to average.

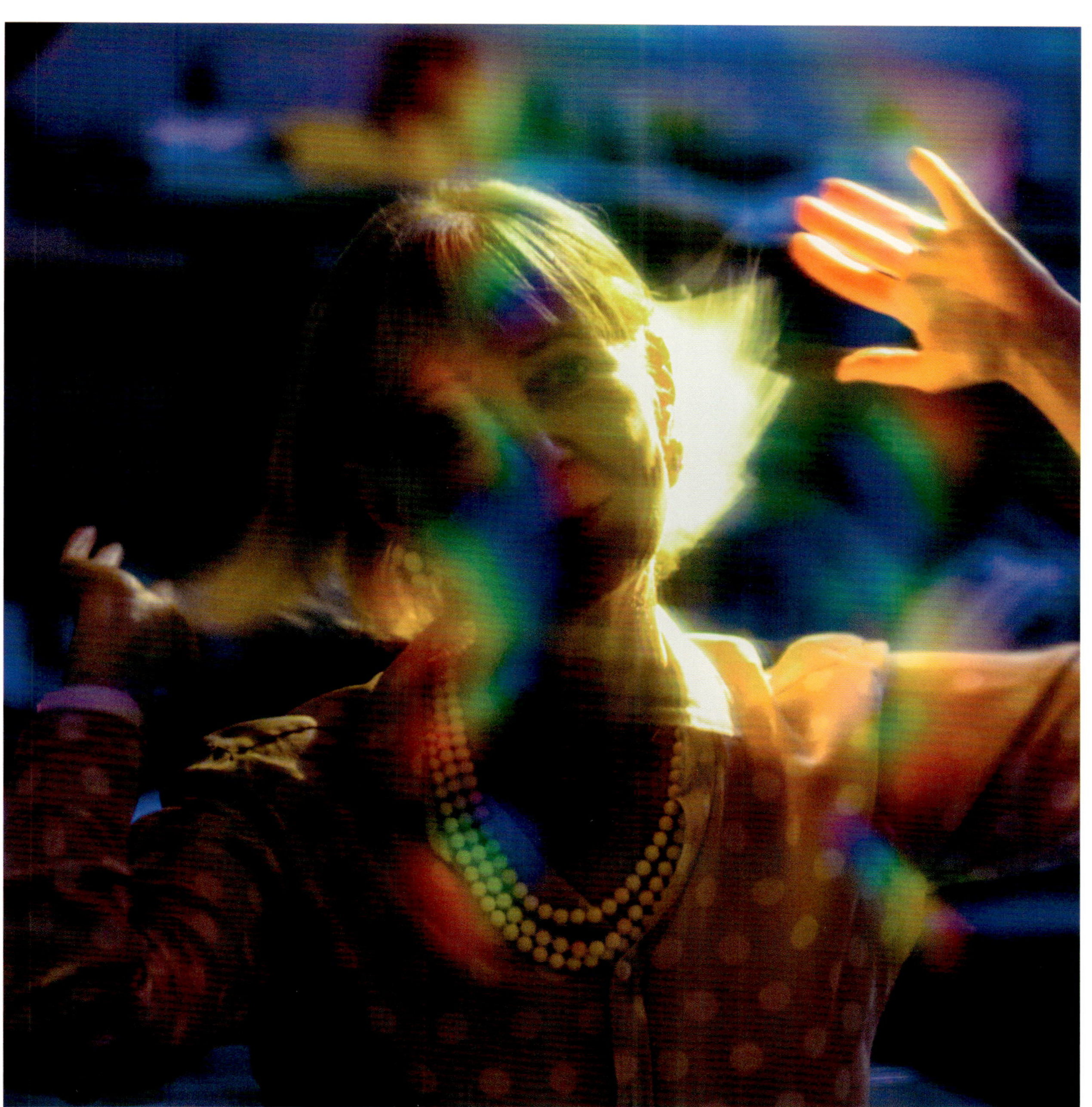

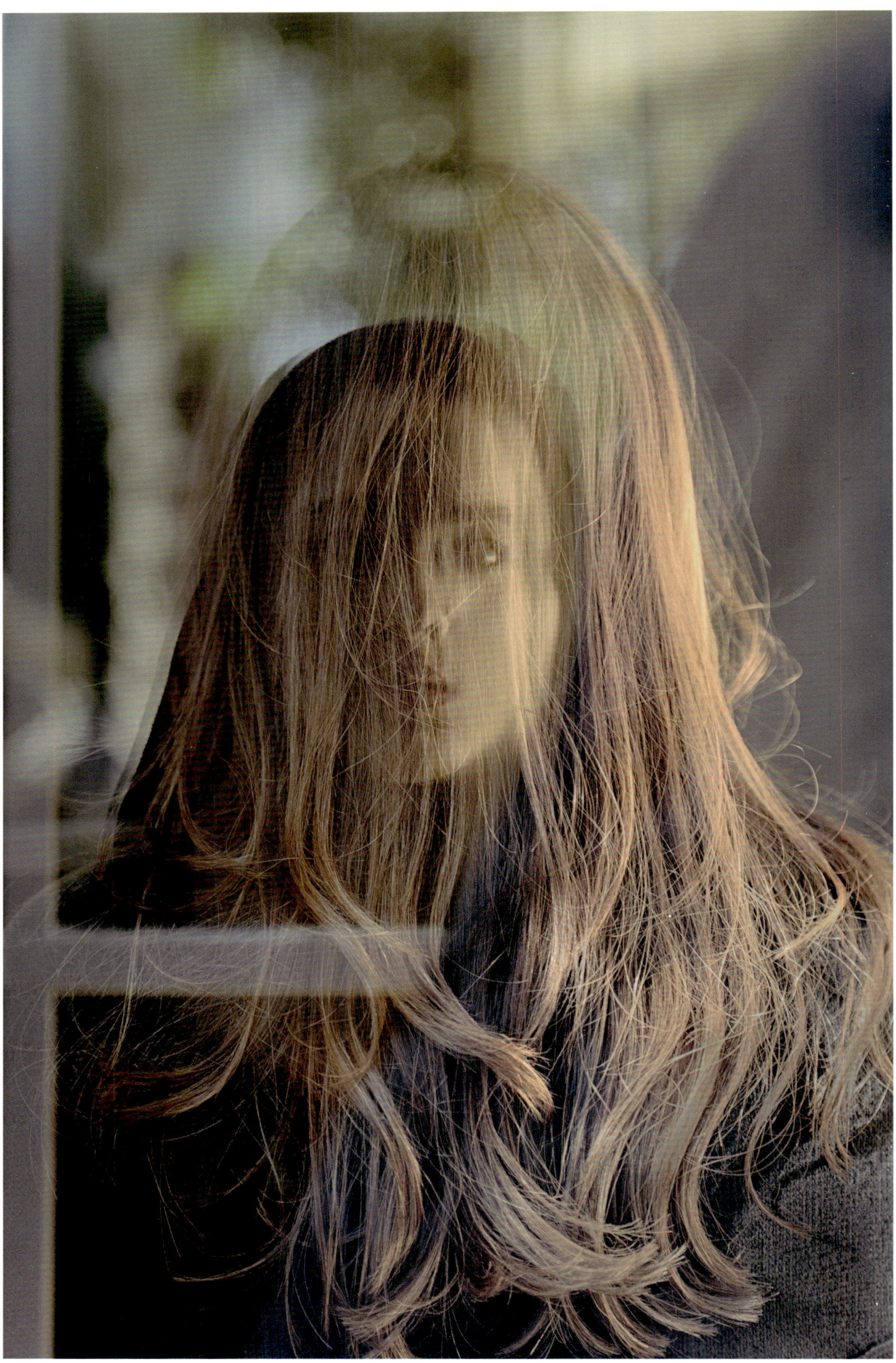

nasha

I took off my jacket, and started unraveling my hijab. I just took it off and thought, "Alright, what else? What else do you want from me?" It felt like I was breaking.

I felt lighter and invisible. That was the best feeling. I didn't have to smile at anybody, and could be pissed off. Whatever I felt inside, I could be. I could blend in, and work on the things that were breaking me. When you wear hijab, there is all this extra stuff you have to worry about: representing Muslims, speaking for Islam, carrying this banner of Islam on your shoulders, and defending and educating people on Islam. It's almost like every girl who wears hijab suddenly has to be a scholar, and explain everything to everyone. You can't just be a girl anymore, going through her own experiences and making her choice.

eliana

I had no issue with covering my hair. It was expected of me as an Orthodox Jewish woman and because I did not yet acknowledge my hair for what it was. I didn't appreciate my hair until I got older. I was looking at pictures over the years and I had gorgeous hair! When I got married I had no issue with covering my hair, because I did not yet appreciate my hair for what it was.

It was through wearing wigs that I realized I had incredible hair; the kind people spend a fortune on. Now that it's been covered for the last five years, it's straight and limp, and no longer has this beautiful coloring. A lot of people would look at that and be saddened by it. For me, though, it's not sad because I'm fulfilling a commandment that God gave me. It brings me closer to God, especially as a divorcée.

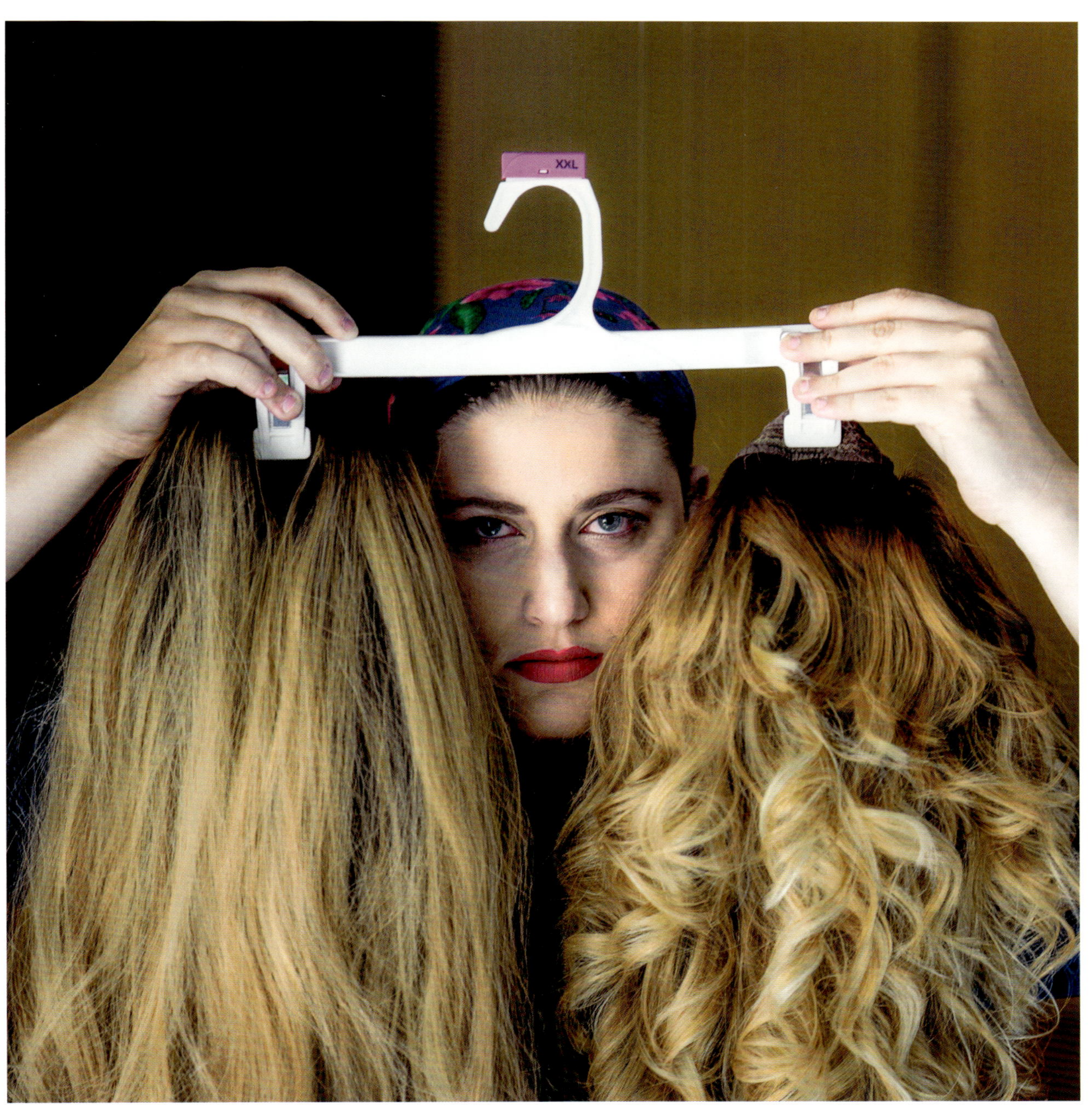
XXL

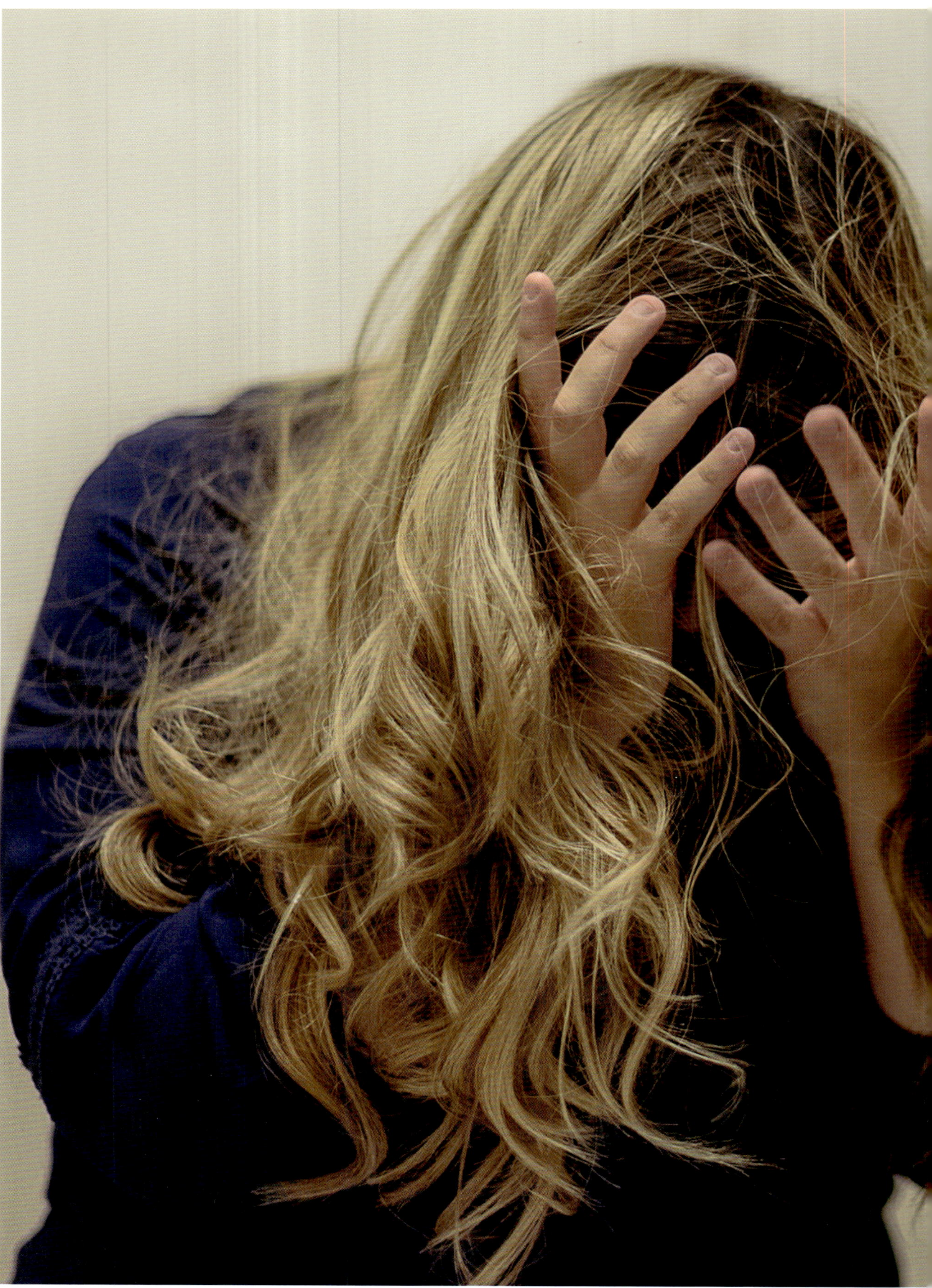

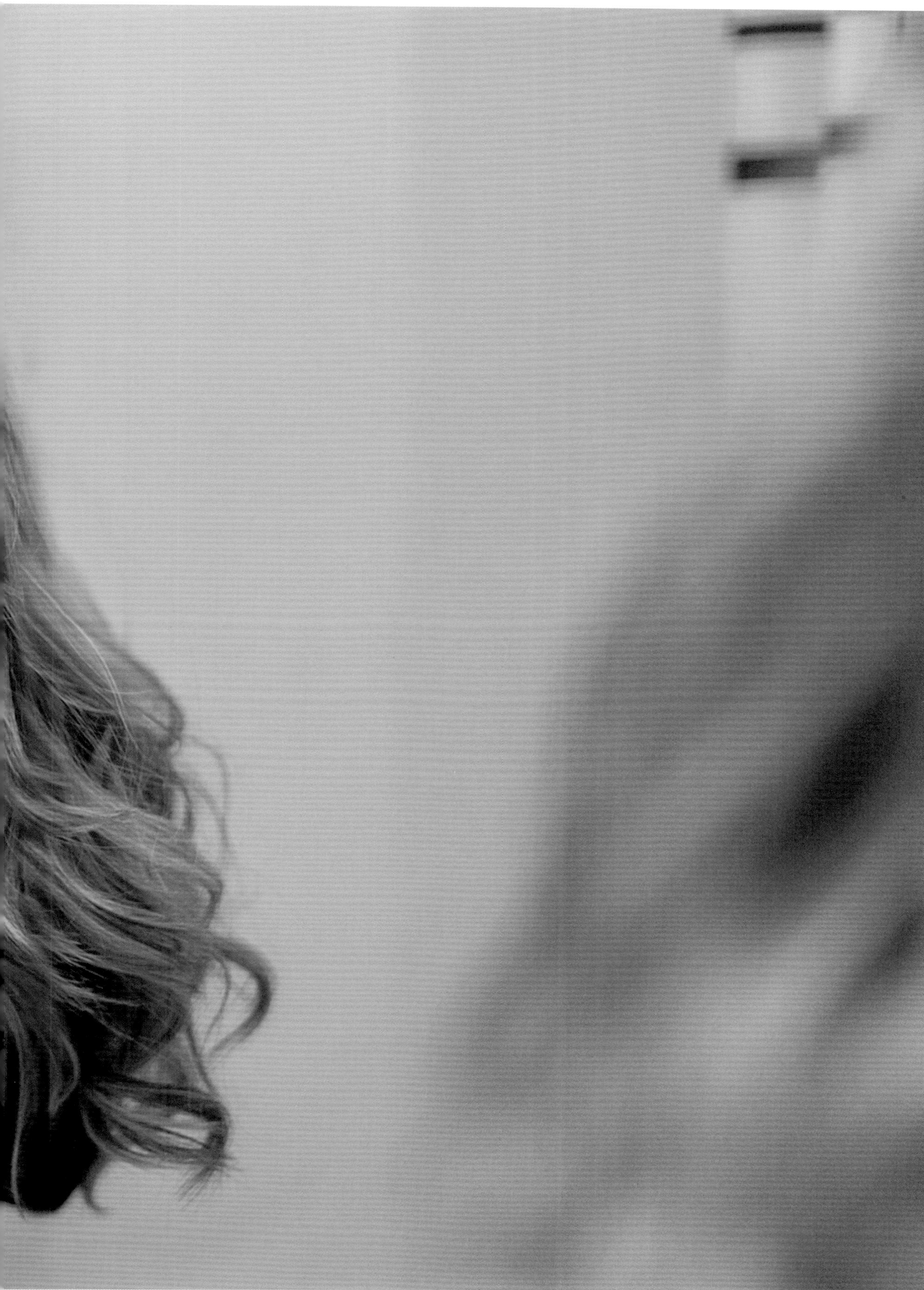

thank you

To my publisher, Damiani, for giving me this opportunity and making my dream a reality.

To all the women that appear in this project, thank you for allowing me to share your stories, your beauty, your truth. This book could not have been made without you. I am forever grateful.

A special thanks to Caleb Cain Marcus for your book design, patience, friendship, and for teaching me all I needed to know about publishing along the way.

A huge thank you to Jonathan Blaustein for believing in me, guiding me from start to finish, helping to edit the copy, and for being an ally throughout.

Thank you to Emily Lambert-Clements for the beautifully written introduction. I am delighted to have you in my life.

To Esther Berry, for the thought-provoking essay, a million thanks. I never thought I would meet someone who is as interested in hair as much as I am!

I am grateful to Aline Smithson, my friend and mentor. Thank you for always sharing so generously your wisdom and love.

Thanks to Ken Merfeld, who taught me all I know about portraiture and whose lessons I bring with me on every shoot.

Thank you to William Bullard who ignited my passion for photography and for giving hours of your free time to teach me when I knew absolutely nothing.

To my dear friend Debra Matlock who worked on editing the audio excerpts for this project and would indulge my outlandish ideas over breakfast, thank you!

Thank you Natasha, Philip, Armando and Eric for making sure that my tech world and printing life worked smoothly. You make me look good. I would be so lost without you!

To my hairdresser Sophie, my friend and confidant for over a decade, thanks for understanding implicitly the importance of hair, and making me feel amazing when I leave your salon.

Thank you to my friends at the Los Angeles Center of Photography that I have leaned on for guidance and advice, for finding me subjects and offering feedback, you are absolutely the best.

The support of my girlfriends has been invaluable to my journey. I thank you with my whole heart.

To my in-laws, Barbara and Stephen, for always being encouraging of my projects and making me feel so lucky and loved.

A huge thank you to my husband David for reading and re-reading every draft of this book and being my partner every step of the way, and my children: Maya, Dillon, and JJ, for all your love and support. Your taking pride in me made it all worthwhile.

Thank you to my sisters, Rinki and Rupali, for allowing me the space to re-visit my past when I needed to but always keeping me grounded in the present.

To my father, Om, thank you for showing me what it means to have courage. And to my mother, Sushma, for teaching me that vulnerability isn't weakness and showing me the way to grace.

HAIR STORIES
ROHINA HOFFMAN

Text has been edited lightly for brevity and clarity.

For audio excerpts of the women's interviews, please visit
womenshairstories.com

Published by Damiani srl
info@damianieditore.com
www.damianieditore.com

Printed in October 2018 by
Grafiche Damiani – Faenza Group SpA, Italy.

ISBN 978-88-6208-640-0

Design & Separations:
Caleb Cain Marcus, Luminositylab.com, New York